THE ART OF
POLARITY
THERAPY

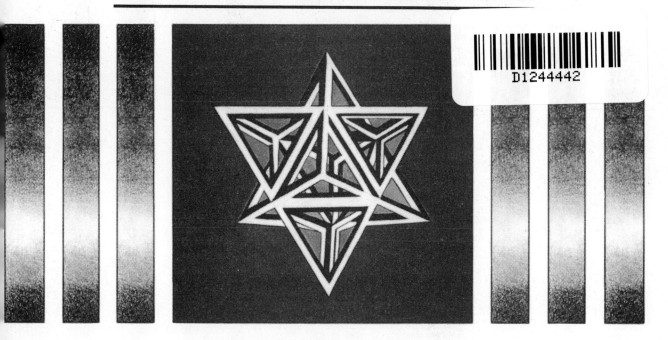

A
PRACTITIONER'S
PERSPECTIVE

Phil Young

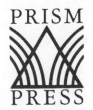

PRISM
PRESS

This book is dedicated to my teacher, Alan Siegel N.D. Thank you Alan for your friendship, understanding, inspiration and support, but most of all thank you for the gift of Polarity Therapy.

THE ART OF POLARITY THERAPY
A Practitioner's Perspective
Published in Great Britain in 1990, 1995 and 2000 by

PRISM PRESS
The Thatched Cottage,
Partway Lane
Hazelbury Bryan,
Sturminster Newton,
Dorset, DT10 2DP

Polarity Therapy balances and stimulates the body's life energy currents. It does not treat or diagnose illness or disease. It is not intended to be a substitute for needed medical care.

Printed in Great Britain by
The Guernsey Press Company Limited, Guernsey, Channel Islands.

Contents

Introduction

This book is in part a very personal statement concerning my own approach to Polarity Therapy as a full-time practitioner and is also a very clear, concise guide to the many techniques that were not included in *Polarity Therapy, the power that heals* written by my teacher Alan Siegel N.D. and myself. If you have not read that book it would be helpful if you did, as it will make this one more accessible, though anyone with a good basic understanding of Polarity Therapy will find this book an invaluable guide to using this fascinating healing art at a professional level. I have structured the book rather like a polarity session beginning with the preliminaries, taking the case history, on through the diagnosis, the energy balancing bodywork and finally reviewing the whole process.

It is a distillation of the knowledge and insight that I have gained since becoming a practising therapist. During this time I have given many thousands of treatments to clients with problems ranging from low back pain to advanced cancerous conditions. For the last three years I have also been running a successful professional training programme in England covering all aspects of polarity therapy. I have also, like most other polarity therapists, spent many a fascinating hour poring over the information-packed, but ultimately confusing books written by the founder of polarity therapy Dr. Randolph Stone. I truly hope this book is a little clearer. I urge you not to give up reading the original books as they contain the experience of many decades of healing work. A level of experience that I cannot match, yet!

At this time (1989) there is a big movement worldwide to establish minimum standards of excellence in the practice of polarity therapy, a move that I heartily applaud and am directly involved in. As Moshe Feldenkrais, the late originator of an amazing technique of movement re-education pointed out before his death, there is no system that has been developed in the realm of somatics that has not been improved upon by the students and practitioners of the system in the following years after the passing of the founder. A sentiment that I am sure Dr. Stone and his named successor Pierre Pannetier would share. Do not be afraid to be creative in your practice. One has only to read Dr. Stone's books to realise that he was a true eclectic who took different parts of many healing arts and blended this knowledge with his own practical experience and unique insight to create Polarity Therapy.

I hope you enjoy studying and applying in your own practice the techniques and insights that I offer in this book and find them as useful as I have. Happy polarising!

1 First Thoughts

In essence all therapy is about creating a relationship with the client that is supportive enough to give them the confidence to heal themselves. All relationships are about contact, communication and change. It has been said that the whole course of a relationship can be charted from the first five minutes of contact between the people involved. If this is true, then in the case of polarity therapy the first few minutes of contact with a client occur most frequently over the telephone. It is important to have some awareness of how to deal with the kind of questions that are raised and to have an ability to present yourself and your work in an appropriate light. The most frequently asked questions are: what is polarity therapy? how does it work? can it help me? how long will it be before I get better? does it work for everyone? are you qualified? There are many other questions that you will be asked but these are the main recurring ones. These questions are often asked during the first actual session, particularly if the issues they concern have not been dealt with in the very first contact. Indeed it is possible to set your practice up in such a way that these issues are only dealt with during the first face-to-face contact, either the first session or during a specific interview created to deal with them. An informatory interview is a particularly good idea if you feel uncomfortable on the telephone.

As a practitioner of polarity therapy do you actually know what you want to achieve in a series of sessions? Is your work orientated towards personal growth, or do you view it as an alternative to allopathic medicine? Do you practise preventative health care and maintenance, or healing in which your hands and energy are superior substitutes for modern drug therapy? Do you do both? Perhaps you see polarity as relaxation therapy for stress release. I can see some purists throwing up their hands in horror at such a thought, yet if some 80 per cent of all illness is caused by stress (a figure which I have noticed goes up every year!) such an approach to polarity therapy can hardly be glibly dismissed. Do you practise it as a form of postural and movement therapy? It is obviously true to say that there is an enormous diversity in the approaches to treatment that a polarity practitioner can offer. The main thing is to know what you do and be able to articulate it in a clear, precise fashion.

In your first contact with a client it is important to communicate with them in terms that they can understand and relate to easily. There is no point in talking about chakras, life energy and the five elements if these terms are not part of the client's vocabulary. There is a need to educate but do not try to begin by getting into deep involved expositions on energy. Develop some very simple explanations about the nature of polarity therapy around terminology that you know everyone is likely to understand, perhaps using such terms as stress, relaxation, good circulation, nervous system stimulation and so on. If you want to talk about energy you can use analogies about flat batteries, magnetism, electrical generating stations, and the national grid. Always begin by speaking to clients in a language they can understand, to create a rapport, then you can start to teach them a new one. To create a secure relationship with a client it is vitally important that they feel they understand the nature of the therapeutic process. It is not important that the explanation you give them is completely accurate, just that it allows them to feel safe, secure and confident.

In some systems of alternative medicine the practitioners are recommended, by the various training establishments, to wear white jackets or overalls whilst giving treatments. I can see why this might have practical value in some therapies but I have always felt that most of my clients were trying to get away from people who wear white coats or uniforms. The clothing you wear whilst giving sessions can have a profound effect on your client. In fact the colour alone could become a form of therapeutic intervention, provided that you have an understanding of the effects of colour upon consciousness and the life energy. If you are going to teach polarity yoga as part of your sessions then your clothing obviously needs to be loose and comfortable, which is fine as long as you know in advance that you intend to do this, but what if it suddenly seems appropriate and you are wearing tight trousers? I finally came to the conclusion that it is important to wear clothing that is comfortable, loose, and smart enough to do anything I wanted to in. I frequently find it useful to put one knee on the bodywork table for support when giving a session and some clothing just does not allow you to do this with dignity — an even greater problem if you wear dresses or skirts. Not that I have actually worn a dress to give a treatment. (Well, that is my story anyway and I am sticking to it!) Seriously though, lady practitioners and my female students have told me they feel the same.

The room you practise in, its decor and ambience can also have a profound effect on your clients. It is ideal if you can set aside a room that is used only for giving treatments. This allows a certain quality of energy to build up in it that is highly beneficial to the healing process. If you have to use a room that is used for other purposes as well, then develop a few simple ways of changing its ambience by doing something other than just setting up a bodywork table. Burn some incense, put up a few charts, whatever will make you feel that it is now a treatment room and not your living room or den. From the client's perspective it will make the whole therapeutic experience more professional, and that is important, certainly in the beginning stages of therapy. At a later date when the relationship is more familiar a relaxed approach is also valuable, as it helps to get away from the 'therapist as god' syndrome that is sometimes cultivated by practitioners, a scenario that is ultimately destructive and de-humanising in my opinion.

When giving a polarity session it has been said that the client should remove all jewellery as the metal has its own effect on the client's energy field; an effect that may be in opposition to the balance you are trying to create in a session. Dr. Stone pointed out many times the powerful effect that gold and silver have on the energy fields, and indeed used these metals extensively in his own practice. I *never* ask a client to take rings off before a session precisely because of the effect of gold and silver on the life energy. I believe that if the effect of these metals is as potent as Dr. Stone indicated, when a client puts the rings back on at the end of the session there will be an instant distortion of the balance that I have so carefully created. I know from my own experience that it is possible to create good balance and flow of life energy when a client is still wearing their jewellery, and that it will not then be a factor that could disrupt the balance that has been achieved after the session. In some cases because of acute energetic sensitivity in general, I have felt it necessary to advise a client to stop wearing jewellery altogether.

4

The amount of metal in a bodywork table can also have a significant effect on your energy balancing work, so the less the better. I also know from my own experience that there is a powerful energy field that emanates from the kind of wood used in a table's construction. I myself asked a master woodworker to create a bodywork table for me, and finally chose beech as the dominant wood in its structure because having scanned many different kinds of wood I felt happiest with its energy quality, although its weight means the table is not portable. I am not saying that beech is *the* wood out of which to make a polarity table but it is the one that suits me best. You may feel differently. It is certainly an area worth exploring if you can, but do not get worried about it if you are not able. Simply get a table you really like even if it is metal and marine plywood. Your positive thoughts will more than compensate. The width of a table is also important, thirty inches wide being a minimum. This can be a problem, particularly in England, where if you are a massage therapist who has trained in polarity therapy at a later date, you will probably already have a table, and standard massage tables here are usually only twenty-four to twenty-six inches wide. You need a table wide enough to allow a client's arms to rest fully relaxed at their sides.

In Polarity Therapy there is a great deal of discussion given to the idea that the practitioner should be 'neutral' when working with clients. What does this actually mean? My own teacher emphasised that because everybody heals at different rates, it was important not to expect to see instant physical results after doing a manipulation as your criteria for success. Pierre Pannetier used to say that we as practitioners do not do anything, it is the life energy that does it all. He also told students to remember that 'You are not the healer'. To me this meant that I did not need to become attached to the results of my treatments. If they worked, that was fine, and if they did not then that was also fine. However, it did seem to me after practising for some time that whilst this had a great deal of benefit for me in that it meant effectively that I never failed regardless of whether a client changed or not, and allowed me to maintain positive feelings concerning my therapeutic skill particularly as this position never called my skills into question, I began to see it as being something less than desirable. I actually became a therapist to facilitate people's self-healing processes, so to adopt a position of neutrality in relation to treatment somehow did not give me a basis upon which to evaluate how good I was. I have always maintained that most, if not all, practitioners of any healing art do it because when they are able to help a client move towards wholeness their egos are given a powerful boost (and their bank balance does not suffer either). There is often a great deal of self deception about why anyone should want to practise as a therapist. When I began to look at my motivations as clearly and honestly as I could, I realised that I did not want to practise from a neutral position, not least because it denied me a certain level of ego satisfaction. I would question any statements from a practitioner to the effect that they did not experience any ego satisfaction from their work, that they only practised for higher or more noble reasons. I myself am a therapist for both selfless, loving, spiritual reasons and much more pragmatic, ego and material needs.

To facilitate the expression of all my reasons for being a therapist, I began to adopt a position in relation to my work that I call 'balanced, positive' as opposed to neutral. In effect, what this means is that I approach polarity therapy with the belief that I am sufficiently skilful to be able to resolve even the most complicated life problems for the client, that I do not expect to see instantaneous healing, but I acknowledge that it can and does occur, so that if a change does not occur for the client I will not consider it a failure on my part, the client's or on the life energy. I will look at it as an opportunity to ascertain in what areas I need to expand my knowledge and skills. It is true that the life energy does everything, but it can only do so when it is flowing freely. My job as a therapist is to make it possible for the life energy to do the healing, and I have found that for me a balanced positive attitude creates the greatest possibility of this occurring. My intention is an extremely powerful, direct yet balanced desire for the client to be able to resolve his problems. An intention that allows me to effect rapid and profound changes in their energy fields.

In Chinese energy theory a great deal of importance is attached to the concept of 'i' and its relationship to 'chi', the Chinese term for life or breath energy. The translation of the Chinese word 'i' is 'mind', 'intent', or sometimes 'mind intent'. The relationship between these two concepts is often expressed as the 'chi' (or energy) flows at the behest of the 'i' or mind intent. To put it another way, your intention, the pattern of your thinking, can control the movement of life energy in your body. It is this law that is fundamental to the effectiveness of nearly all self-healing visualisations and affirmations. As polarity therapists this fact has enormous significance in that it is your mind intent, or to put it more simply your intention, that controls the quality and kind of energetic interaction that occurs between you and your client.

The greater the clarity of thought and intention that you bring to your sessions the more effective your treatments will become. When I began practising polarity therapy one of the first things that I became interested in was whether I was sufficiently sensitive to be able to differentiate between the different elemental energies in a client's energy field. At first I did feel that I was able to tell which quality of energy I was interacting with at any time. Then I began to notice that if I had evaluated a client as having a particular kind of elemental imbalance, then that was always the quality of energy that I interacted with during the bodywork. Quite frankly after a while I really began to wonder how it was that I always seemed to get it right! How was I always able to deduce before a treatment began what elements were out of balance? Particularly when some of the treatments did not create any significant change in the client's condition. Most obviously I was not always right! I then began to experiment with making clearly false-to-fact evaluations concerning the particular energetic imbalances that a client was manifesting, and working on that basis. I worked in the full belief that the evaluation that I made was the correct one. What happened was that the energy I predominantly interacted with was always the one that I had falsely decided to be the problem. It began to seem more and more that the concept that energy follows thought was true not just in terms of controlling your own energy flows and in the process of self healing, but it also applied in my interaction with the client's energy. These and other experiences showed me just how powerful a practitioner's intention is in determining both the quality and function of their energy release work.

In polarity therapy the most active way of communicating with the client is through physical touch or, more correctly, energetic touch. Dr. Stone defined three types of touch that can be used in polarity therapy. To use the sanskrit terminology they are rajasic, satvic, and tamasic. Roughly translated these types of touch could be called, respectively: stimulating, balancing and dispersing. There is something of a split or schism amongst practitioners of polarity therapy concerning the relative value of the tamasic quality of touch. However, before we look at this in more detail a deeper look at each kind of touch as defined by Dr. Stone is appropriate.

RAJASIC

The function of rajasic or stimulating touch is to move energy. To stir it up. It is done with a positive but light hand contact that moulds itself to the contours of the body. The hand is then vibrated, moved backwards and forwards or in circular fashion, so that the movement which occurs is the skin moving over the underlying tissue. In other words, the hand does not slide over the skin but stays in the same place. Depending on the amplitude and range of your movement the client's body may go into oscillation, a gentle rocking motion. This kind of touch resonates with the outward or centrifugal movement of energy in the client's body, the energy flow as it moves from the core of the energy field to the circumference. It is a positively charged contact.

SATVIC

The function of satvic or balancing touch is to calm the energy, to bring it into balance, to smooth its flow so that there is no turbulence. It is done with a very light touch that moulds itself gently to the contour of the body. There is no intentional physical movement involved. This kind of touch resonates with all the neutrally charged areas of the body, the central axes, and the areas where the energy currents cross over creating perfect balance, specifically the chakras and the joints. It is a neutrally charged contact.

TAMASIC

The function of the tamasic or dispersing touch is to break up chronic energy blocks within the body's energy field. It is done with a deep penetrating touch that goes down into the underlying tissues beneath the contact area. It is a deep tissue technique that seeks to release the energy locked in areas of extreme muscular tension, areas where the physical tension is impeding the flow of energy, blood, lymph and nutrients, where there is a lot of accumulated toxicity and poor drainage. It releases energy so that it can complete its return flow from the circumference back to the core of the energy field, the centripetal flow of energy. It is a negatively charged contact.

All polarity therapists use the rajasic and satvic touches, but only some use the tamasic touch as well. Pierre Pannetier, the successor to Dr. Stone, emphasised the lighter rajasic and satvic work on the basis that people in pain are already hurting enough, so what justification was there for adding to it? Even Dr. Stone says in his writings that patients do not easily forgive you for inflicting pain on them, and that when giving a treatment you should be gentle. He also recommends deep work and heavy pressure release. If we look at the basis of his reasoning for using a deep tamasic touch it is in essence that a blockage manifesting as a congestion in the muscle tissue indicates a lack of circulation, and that the key to releasing this is to drain the muscle of toxins and fluids by deep pressure which will squeeze the stagnant fluids out, creating a vacuum effect, a space that will be filled by fresh blood and prana that will facilitate the detoxification process. Energetically it is also true that opposites attract in the centripetal flow of energy and that like charges repel, so by using a negatively charged touch on a blocked area with a negative charge, there is a repelling effect that will push the blocked energy back to its source, releasing the flow. This process almost always induces real soreness for a period of time until the last of the toxins are cleared, all of which is indicative of the energy currents moving again. This I know through my own experimentation with tamasic touch to be perfectly valid. However, I have also discovered that it is not necessary. It is quite possible to release these stagnant areas by using the rajasic touch and even the satvic touch as defined by Dr. Stone.

Dr. Stone says in his writings that the key to releasing blockages at the congested negative

7

poles is 'stimulation'. The tamasic work is extremely stimulating and creates very fast results and a lot of discomfort. The rajasic touch is also stimulating. The key to making it effective on very congested areas is to find the right *direction of application* that releases the energy. The end result is the same. The toxins are cleared and the energy flows freely again, but the difference is that it takes a little longer and it is a lot less painful. The time difference, in my experience, is that if a tamasic treatment is going to clear the system it takes between twenty-four and forty-eight hours, whereas a rajasic treatment will take some two to four days, a totally negligible difference in my opinion. There is also a possibility that you can release too much toxicity into the client's system all at once, and create secondary problems if their eliminative system is already overloaded. This is a serious point that you should consider in all your work, particularly if you are working with cancerous conditions. It is quite possible to break up tumours using energy-based techniques, polarity or otherwise. Always make sure the eliminative system is functioning well enough to deal with the massive amount of debris that can be dumped into the system during the healing process.

It is also possible to release deep congestion with satvic touch. This can be done in two ways. Firstly, using the fact that life energy flows from your right to your left hand, you can easily bring increasing amounts of energy into the blocked area by placing your left hand on it and having your right hand on the positive pole of the particular area, and waiting until you feel the energy reacting very strongly beneath your left hand. Once this is happening simply reverse your hands and send the energy back to its supply pole, the positive pole. You have now created a powerful complete flow of life energy through the blocked area, which will clear the congestion. It is also possible to extend this technique to include the negative pole of the blocked area. The other way, which simply involves holding the blocked area, is based upon the fact that the polarity of these deeply blocked areas is negative and that it is the inward or return flow of energy that is blocked. In this phase of energy movement 'opposites attract', and as a satvic touch is in effect an opposite charge to the blocked area (remember that positive and negative are relative terms, so a neutrally charged touch is still positive in relation to a blocked area that is negatively charged), you will in effect attract the energy block towards your contact hand, regardless of whether it is your right or left hand, as long as it is acting as a satvic neutrally charged contact. As you move the blockage out of its original position, fresh prana will instantly begin to flow in and through that area again. At the moment the energy block, the stagnant prana, moves it has to break up and disperse because its static nature has changed. It is moving again, and if it is moving it is no longer by definition blocked energy, so it has to dissipate back into the overall economy of the body's energy field. This particular energetic process also occurs when using rajasic touch because of the polarities involved. In terms of the time these satvic releases take to work, in my experience, they seem to follow some logic all of their own. Sometimes the change seems almost instantaneous with even the physical tension, and at other times it takes four or five days. I have never been able to discover a discernible pattern.

Some practitioners have expressed the opinion that the 'light' work is too slow, but I have never been able to get a satisfactory answer as to how they define 'slow' in relation to energy work as being a pejorative. I hardly think that the difference of a few days or even a couple of weeks, can be thought of as a valid objection to the effectiveness of the light work. From the client's point of view the main consideration is often quick relief from pain. The rajasic and satvic work is no less effective than the tamasic work in this area in relation to time, as there is always a significant reduction in pain *immediately*. It is the full resolution that just takes that much longer. In fact, I have some doubts that a full resolution ever truly occurs when the tamasic work is used extensively. My own personal experience of working on clients who have been treated by practitioners whose approach uses a lot of deep tamasic work, is that the energy blocks are often pushed deeper into the system. What has happened is that as I have worked gently on areas that have apparently been resolved of energetic disturbance by other practitioners, the original problem has reappeared in full force. To me this indicates a deep suppression of the imbalance as opposed to a proper resolution. I can from my own personal experience of tamasic work see how this might occur, in that if pain is indicative of blocked energy, and if energetically there is a contraction in any problem area, then increasing the pain by deep work can simply cause greater contraction at a deeper level. It also seems possible that it may cause the blockage to be pushed so deep that it enters into the mind energy field and becomes, to use Dr. Stone's terminology, a sensory energy block. One that is too fine to show up in any structural disturbance.

You have only to experience deep tamasic work on yourself to realise the degree of mental-emotional withdrawal that is a natural response to the pain it creates. As energy follows thought this is the last thing you want to occur when trying to resolve disturbances in the energy fields. Encouraging the client to go into the pain rather than withdraw from it is a useful technique to use when doing tamasic work, but unfortunately unless the client has a high degree of masochism in their make up they will only go into the pain with a portion of their conscious awareness. A full release can only occur when both conscious and unconscious awareness is involved totally. As one of the functions of the unconscious mind is protection, then even though there may be a conscious sense of going into the pain, the unconscious is quite likely to be watching the therapist and saying something internally like 'what do you think I am, stupid or something? You are the one causing most of the pain, and you want me to experience it more!'.

As a descriptive metaphor let us look at water and its behaviour as a good analogy for energetic processes. In any blocked area we could typify the blockages as being ice. To allow the water to flow freely the ice must be removed. This could be done in one of two ways: either tamasically by hitting it and breaking it up, or rajasic/satvically by melting it with the heat of your hands. In the former the ice will certainly break up, allowing the water to flow again, but what about the shards of ice that would get smashed into the surrounding structure in the process? What about the damage caused to the surrounding structure by the original impact? What about the fragments that are released? Perhaps some are still too big to break up naturally and flow freely through the whole system, necessitating your having to follow them around breaking them up when they get stuck. A time consuming process! Whereas, in the latter case, the icy blockage just melts, becoming water again and allowing free flow with no damage to the surrounding area and no likelihood of it causing a blockage elsewhere. I know the scenario I would prefer to create if this analogy has any validity.

Before moving on from our exploration of the three 'classic' kinds of polarity contacts, as defined by Dr. Stone, if we go back to his definitions of the different kinds of touch it is obvious that there is both a physical component to each touch and an energetic component. It is possible to create at least nine different kinds of touch by combining these components in different ways. The physical component of rajasic touch is a firm surface contact that moves tissues beneath the skin. Satvic touch is very light surface contact only, with little or no movement. Tamasic touch is deep sub-surface contact achieved by strong pressure, and can be done with or without movement. As movement is a variable quality in each kind of touch, leaving it aside as a consideration the physical parameters we are left with are contacts that are surface, just below surface and deep into the structure. The energetic component of rajasic touch is its positive charge that increases the outflow of energy, of satvic touch it is its neutral charge that balances, and of tamasic touch it is its negative charge that sends the currents back to their source. Dr. Stone typified the positive outflow of energy as warm and creative, the negative inflow as cool and constructive, and the neuter source and its reflection at the most expansive point of the outflow (and beginning of the inflow) as stillness. Energetically I like to think that the positive charged touch says 'let's go and play', the neutral charged touch says 'let's rest and relax awhile', and the negatively charged touch says 'let's go home'. I used these and other relevant images as ways of attuning my conscious intention to arouse the energy currents as specifically as possible.

This gives the possibility of nine different types of touch, as set out below, all creating quite different effects.

PHYSICAL	ENERGETIC
1. Surface Touch	Neutral Charge
2. Below Surface	Neutral Charge
3. Deep Touch	Neutral Charge
4. Surface Touch	Positive Charge
5. Below Surface	Positive Charge
6. Deep Touch	Positive Charge
7. Surface Touch	Negative Charge
8. Below Surface	Negative Charge
9. Deep Touch	Negative Charge

Physical movement or lack of it could be added to the model, creating further permutations. The classic rajasic touch would be a no.5 type touch, the satvic contact a no.1 type touch, and the tamasic contact a no.9 type touch. It is clear that there is a way of modulating the classical tamasic contact so that you can clear congested tissues but without undue pain, and also that you can do tamasic work on the surface of the body. All you need is the right intention. From your reading of the aforegoing it might have seemed that I never do deep tamasic work, but the truth is I use it all the time. It is just that I do it from the surface and allow my energy to reach the appropriate depth, which is a relatively painless experience for the client. I trust the energy to do the work necessary to clear blockages. I decided a long time ago that to use negatively charged contacts and to feel that I had to go physically deep into the tissues simply meant that I really did not trust the life force, or that the quality of my intention had anything to do with the process. The release of energy blocks by using surface lever contacts and modulating the polarities, touches 1, 4, and 7, is, from my experience, a relatively painless process for the client apart from the occasionally intense sensations that occur as the blockage lets go. Detoxification happens at a natural rate that is easily supported by the client's eliminative capacity.

It is my opinion that there is nothing that can be achieved by the tamasic work as described by Dr. Stone that cannot be achieved by far more gentle methods. I suspect his work was enormously influenced by his original training in the physical techniques of chiropractic and osteopathy, some of which, as I know from personal experience, are quite ferocious. It is a tribute to his sensitivity and creativity that he was able to change his work from the physical to the energetic. I understand he also said that all students of polarity therapy should read and study his books and then move on from there. In this day and age when there are so many incredibly subtle energy-based techniques being developed, I cannot help but wonder about the personality of practitioners who use a lot of deep painful work on their clients. Is it just that they have a certain sadistic streak or a lot of blocked fire energy that they are trying to work through at their client's expense? Deep tamasic work can be very confrontational, and whilst there are perhaps occasions when confrontation is valid, as a general practice I do not see how it can be justified. Interestingly you can get a lot of emotional release from deep tamasic work, but unfortunately it is not really the kind of spontaneous release that can be so important in a client's movement towards health. It is basically an emotional response to pain. We can all cry and be upset when we are feeling physical pain, but it is just a response, not the expression of a causative factor. I have heard it argued that it can help a person to release their fire energy, but the chances of a client with a fire problem being able to confront the powerful position the therapist occupies is not perhaps impossible but is highly unlikely. If you have picked up the message during your polarity training that emotional release is an important part of the therapeutic process you were probably taught well. However, if you think that deep tamasic work is a way of fulfilling this requirement then you are on the wrong track. What you need to do is refine your intention and your energetic sensitivity so that you are spontaneously drawn to the places in the client's energy field where the emotions are being held. All you need to do then is make a contact with the energy, create some movement and the emotions will come up. At that point remember the golden rule, *Do Not Panic*, just be there with them and allow it to change.

There are a few important points that you should bear in mind if you decide that you want to use the classic version of tamasic touch. Pressure applied to an area is a force acting at right angles to the contact surface. If you do not apply the force at right angles to the contact surface you will bring into play frictional forces. Working on someone's spine using a strong tamasic touch you should apply the force at right-angles to the surface of the skin. This is particularly important if you are working over the transverse processes of a vertebra. Should you apply the force at any other angle than at right angles to the flat surface of the transverse process you will create friction and shearing stresses in relation to the other bones. This is very painful for the client and is potentially dangerous, as should the forces become too great it is quite possible that you might damage the bone structure. These factors are even more critical if you use your elbow to do deep tissue work. However, this is not to say that you should never apply force at any other angle than right angles to the contact surface. You should be aware that when you do so the amount of pressure put on a particular area immediately increases because the diagonal force consists of two components, the amount of pressure acting at right angles plus the additional frictional force that in effect prevents your hand from sliding off the contact area.

When doing any kind of rajasic work that involves rocking the body you should be aware that any body that is made to oscillate has a natural frequency. This frequency is determined by the body's mass in relation to the axis around which it is moving. As an example, a simple pendulum will swing quickly with a short length of string and the same pendulum will swing more slowly the longer the string gets. What this means in relation to a rajasic rocking movement that brings a client's whole body into oscillation is that it will be relatively of a much lower frequency than should you be rocking one leg from the hip. The natural frequency, for whichever section of the body you are rocking, is the rhythm that is maintained with the least amount of added force. This is easily felt because you will be able to maintain that rhythm with little effort. It is the same principle that applies when you are pushing a child on a swing. At a certain point you will be able to maintain their swinging movement with just a very small additional push every now and then.

Rajasically stimulating the body as a whole or any particular part, at its natural frequency, nearly always gets the best energetic release possible. Just as in pushing a child on a swing, you do not follow the child as it swings continually pushing, you actually wait for the swing to come back to you before applying the next push. When rocking the body you do not follow the movement continually forcing the frequency, you allow the elasticity of the body to bring it back into your hand, having completed a cycle of movement before applying the next push. Should you apply the next push too soon or too late you will either change the frequency to one other than the natural one or you will stop the oscillation altogether. Working at the natural frequency is relatively effortless and this allows you to very easily sense any changes in the amount of force needed to maintain the oscillation. This is useful in that you can instantly sense any shifts in the tension patterns and energetic balance of a particular body area. It can occasionally be difficult to find the natural frequency, either because a client is actively trying to help the movement, or because sometimes the movement is masked by tension patterns in other areas of the body. Generally speaking, after rocking for a short while any interference eases and you can then pick up the natural frequency.

2   Taking the Case History

Taking a client's case history is basically an in-depth information gathering process. The greater the clarity you have concerning the nature of a client's problems and their etiology, the more likely you are to be able to create effective therapeutic interventions. Taking the case history is definitely linked to your overall diagnosis. The basic skill necessary for taking an accurate case history is to be able to listen, but no less important is your visual perception. The skill of listening encompasses not just hearing what the client has to say, but knowing the right questions to ask that will elicit the most relevant information.

The most fundamentally important questions to ask when taking a case history are what, how, where and when. You are basically trying, in the first phase of information gathering, to define the actual nature of the client's problem. The very first question that I ask a client is 'How can I help you?' The questions that you ask after this first question are always aimed towards clarifying their answer. In fact this is an ongoing process, each new question that you ask is always to clarify the preceding answer. The usage of your visual skill comes into play whilst the client is answering your questions. Basically you are watching their body language as they answer. Are they tense, are they relaxed, how are they sitting, what kind of hand gestures are they making, are their legs or feet moving? Your visual field of perception needs to be wide enough to encompass their whole body. To do this you must not sit too close to the client, so give some forethought to the layout of your treatment room. The reason that the client's body language is so important is that it allows you to access information in relation to your questions that the client is not consciously aware of, because all body language is generated by the client's sub-conscious mind. For example, suppose you ask a client about the quality of their intimate personal relationships and their reply to this is that they are fine and that they have no problems in this area, yet as they give this verbal response their body suddenly becomes tense or agitated; this could lead you to believe that in spite of what they said there was definitely some problem in this area, or, to use a Polarity term, that there was a 'charge' associated with this subject. We could say that you are experiencing an incongruity between the client's words and their body language. In fact, picking up on incongruent statements in relation to previous statements or body language is perhaps the most important aspect in obtaining a valid case history. It is important to remember that it is quite common for a client to lie to you without realising that they are doing so because their own awareness of their problems is often limited. Any time you pick up an incongruity, at whatever level, always explore that area from another angle either there and then or at a later date. In your further questioning do not ever accuse the client of lying because what you are really dealing with is either sub-conscious suppression or self deception. We are all prone to manifesting these processes, which are fundamentally protective in nature.

Unless you have a truly phenomenal memory you are going to have to make notes as you take the case history, either in great detail or at least noting the most salient points. The ability to maintain an uninterrupted flow of conversation whilst at the same time taking notes is essential. Sometimes it is useful to create a standardised case history form that you can fill out for each new client. Such a form would have a space for the client's name, address, date of birth, presenting problem, medication, previous illnesses, previous treatment, diet, sleep patterns, leisure pursuits, occupation, marital status, children and so on. The actual areas that the form covers would be those areas that you feel are most important in relation to how you work. Such a form can also have a space for writing down the actual treatments that you give, and can become an important record for insurance purposes.

At the beginning in taking a case history most of the information exchanged revolves around what is called the 'presenting illness'. The presenting illness is quite often not the real problem that has to be dealt with but is only the surface level of imbalance. It is the problem area that is most familiar to the client but which is often only an effect not an actual cause. Very often the presenting illness will have a label or name given to it by the client's doctor, or sometimes by another alternative medical practitioner. If that is so make a note of it and then dismiss it from your consciousness. If it is a named disease that you are not familiar with then by all means look it up in a medical dictionary, but remember polarity therapy deals with energetic imbalances not physical diseases. What you really want to know is exactly how a particular named presenting illness affects them physically, mentally, emotionally.

If a client comes to you and says that they have arthritis of the knee, all that actually tells you is that a doctor has given them a label for their problem. It tells you nothing about how they experience the arthritis. Diseases are always individual even though broadly speaking it may be possible to label them by defining certain features common to a wide range of symptoms. The kind of things you need to know when trying to ascertain a client's individual experience of a particular problem are: is it a constant experience or does the pain or awareness of the imbalance vary throughout the day? does it vary over a period of a week? what does any pain they experience actually feel like? is it hot, cold, sharp, dull, etc? Always try and get as much detail as possible concerning their particular problem.

Having looked at the presenting illness in depth it is important to then begin working back through all a client's past illnesses. You should look at the recent past of the last few years, but sometimes it is relevant to go as far back as their early childhood. What you are trying to do here is obtain a broad picture of all their past problems, how long they lasted, the kind of treatment they received and so forth. What you are looking for is a pattern of imbalances over the years. Sometimes you will also discover the causative factor of their current problems. I once had a client who came with abdominal distention and constipation which had been a problem for a number of years, which was, I suspect, initially triggered by having a difficult pregnancy some seven years previously. She had become anaemic, been given large doses of iron and became very constipated as a result. Her body, it seemed, had never properly recovered from the side effects of the treatment she received for the anaemia.

Once you have built up a picture of a client's current and previous state of health, you need to get some sense of the kind of life they lead. Are they married? do they have children? what sort of work do they do? what do they do in their spare time? what do they do to relax? are they satisfied with their life as a whole? what are the problem areas? All these questions and many others are useful in trying to come to some understanding of the kind of life a client leads. One area that can be very useful to explore is that of any major breaks in a client's life; by that I mean the death of relatives or other important people, change of occupation, moving house, divorce or separation, birth of children or a child leaving home. All these particular points in a person's life are extremely stressful and can have an enormous effect on their wellbeing. Do not be surprised if a client seems somewhat inarticulate when it comes to talking about themselves; it may be the first time anyone has actually asked them these kind of questions.

After getting a picture of the client's life style, the next important area is to find out what kind of diet they eat. The simplest way to do this is to ask them to go through a typical day's food consumption, describing what they eat at each meal. Apart from checking what they eat at main meal times find out if they eat between meals. Ask them about their daily fluid intake, how much and what it is, and do not forget that such phrases as 'four cups of coffee a day' are relatively meaningless as the size of cups varies enormously. There is a great deal of difference between instant and espresso coffee. Make sure that you obtain precise answers. Do not forget to check alcohol intake. If you have not already done so this is a good point at which to check on what kind of drugs they take, not just prescription ones for particular problems but drugs like aspirin, paracetamol or 'recreational' drugs. An up-to-date dictionary of drugs is of invaluable help when trying to sort out what the possible effects and side effects of the drugs might be. Keep watching the client's body language!

The amount of time needed to take a case history can vary from fifteen minutes to around three-quarters of an hour. It really depends upon how articulate the client is about their particular problems. Sometimes, I have felt that I would have been more successful trying to get blood out of a stone than getting some basic case history information out of certain clients. It is important to remember that if a client has been 'trained' in the procedures of orthodox medicine, then the whole alternative wholistic approach to health care can be quite a shock. Effectively your first job, apart from getting a full case history, is to educate them in wholistic health care and preventative medicine.

It is important to realise that the process of taking a case history becomes an ongoing process as the client continues in therapy. At the beginning of each session a portion of time is always spent in review. One of the first questions that I ask at the beginning of each session is 'Tell me what has happened since I last saw you', or something similar. At this point you need to know what changes have occurred before you can proceed with treatment. Many of the questions that you asked in taking your first case history will still be relevant, and the answers you get will in all probability be different. The time needed to obtain the updated case history is nearly always much less than the original, perhaps only ten to fifteen minutes. Occasionally it can take nearly as long, particularly if the client feels happier and more confident about the nature of the work you are doing. It can be surprising what you learn during the second session.

Ultimately taking a good case history depends upon your ability to get a client to open up and express themselves freely. This is dependent upon the amount of rapport that you can establish with them. To create a good rapport between yourself and a client is to establish a relationship with them in which they can feel safe and secure. A feeling of security is vital to the free flow of what is often quite intimate and personal information. The process of creating a good rapport with a client depends on many factors but they can all be encapsulated in the concept of 'resonance'. Resonance is one of the most important concepts in Polarity Therapy. It comes into play in all areas of treatment, from taking the case history to the energy balancing bodywork.

When two vibrating objects whose fundamental or basic frequency is the same are brought together they will resonate. When two objects resonate the volume or amplitude of the particular frequency at which they vibrate will increase enormously. They are then said to form a resonating system. However, in the first instance should one of the objects not be vibrating, then as the other actively vibrating object is brought towards it it will force or entrain a response in the inactive object, making it vibrate at the same frequency, and then they will be able to resonate together as a system. The classic example of this is the school physics experiment used to demonstrate the principle of resonance and entrainment, in which two tuning forks of the same frequency are used to represent the resonating system. Holding a tuning fork in each hand you tap one of the forks firmly against a hard surface to set it vibrating at its natural frequency, and then bring it slowly towards the other fork. At a certain distance apart the non-vibrating fork will suddenly begin to vibrate as the vibrating fork forces or entrains it to respond. They are then vibrating in harmony and are in resonance.

The principle of resonance applies to any vibrating objects. The human body and its energy field most definitely constitute a vibrating object, and any two or more people can constitute a resonating system. Indeed, because of the complexity of the human body, mind and energy system it can even be said to form a resonating system within itself. Much of the actual energy maps and balancing techniques are based upon this principle. If you understand the physics of music and the concept of harmonics you understand the basis of polarity therapy. When giving a polarity treatment it is obvious that the practitioner and client constitute a resonating system. The client, because of their pain and illness, would be the inactive, non-vibrating part of the system; the therapist the active vibrating part who will entrain a similar response in the client, thereby effectively helping the client to return to full health. This concept gives us another definition of health in relation to human beings. To be healthy is to vibrate fully at your natural frequency.

This principle should not put you off giving a treatment when you are not feeling good, because in the human being it is predominantly the energy that is responsible for the resonance, and the state of your energy is ultimately controlled by your mind or consciousness. Giving a treatment is one of the best ways I know of becoming one-pointed in your consciousness and freeing your energy. The other point about a resonating system is that it is a reciprocal or two-way process. You could say that every time you give a polarity treatment you receive a polarity treatment.

The process of resonance begins with the first true contact that you have with the client, the first session. Taking the case history is really the first opportunity that you have to do anything of a practical nature towards the process of entrainment. As I mentioned earlier the term for this process during the case history taking is 'rapport'. To create a good rapport with a client involves the process of pacing, which itself has two main elements, matching and mirroring.

In essence pacing is a technique for entering the client's reality. In practice this means that you should pay attention to the kind of language structure and content that the client uses, and modify your own to something similar. You are then matching their style of communication. This will ensure that the client has the best possible chance of under-standing both your questions and any information of an educational nature that you might want to share with them. I touched on this concept in the previous chapter when discussing the kind of difficulties involved in explaining to a client exactly what polarity therapy is and how it works. However, matching does more than simply improve communication.It subtly creates a commonality of experience between you and the client, and this makes it very much easier for you to understand the nature of their problems. It is a mistake to believe that we all inhabit the same world. There are in fact something like four billion different ones in total, here on one quite small planet.

Mirroring is basically making your body posture and gestures a mirror of the client's own. This is a natural phenomena that occurs all the time in our everyday lives. Just watch two strangers on a park bench sometime and you will see that after a while they will mirror each other's positions. In the therapeutic environment such mimicry should be done subtly, otherwise if you make what you are doing too obvious the client will feel that you are making fun of them. Another aspect to mirroring is to allow yourself to become aware of the client's breathing rhythm and match your own to it. This particular form of matching is very powerful, as it is moving in to the realm of energetic matching which can create a profound change in the client's state of consciousness. The overall process of pacing is done by any good therapist more or less unconsciously, regardless of whether they have any understanding of the concept. Now that you have an understanding of the concept just watch yourself with a part of your awareness the next time you give someone a polarity session to see when you are actually doing it. I can guarantee that you do it some of the time. Simply notice when you do it and have the thought that it will happen more often. Trying to force yourself to use pacing all the time tends to create a rather gross quality to what should be, and in normal everyday experience is, a subtle phenomena. Creating good rapport should be something that happens as easily as breathing and with as little attention. Allowing something to happen, once you have an understanding of it, is the best way to utilise new information. Very often 'trying' to do something seems to invoke the psychological equivalent of Newton's third law of motion that states 'for every action there is an equal and opposite reaction'.

One other tool that can be very useful in taking the case history is a five element check list. Basically this is a sheet of paper with the various elements and their functions listed in tabular form with small boxes, beside each category, for you to tick if the client has a disturbance in that particular area or function. A sample checklist is reproduced here (Fig. 1). It is by no means a definitive version and I suggest you create your own. I have found them very useful in creating a visual model of a client's imbalances. It allows you to see at a glance when fully filled out where the predominant disturbance is. In the sample chart you would tick the box if there was any kind of disturbance for that area but you could use other parameters of your own choosing to create a more specific representation.

Elemental Checklist
Name: **Date of Birth:**

Ether	*Air*	*Fire*	*Water*	*Earth*
Joints ☐	Shoulders ☐	Eyes ☐	Breasts ☐	Neck ☐
	Kidneys ☐	Solar p. ☐	Genitals ☐	Bowels ☐
	Ankles ☐	Thighs ☐	Feet ☐	Knees ☐
Hearing ☐	Touch ☐	Vision ☐	Taste ☐	Smell ☐
Throat ☐	Chest ☐	Head ☐	Pelvis ☐	Abdomen ☐
	Circulation ☐	Vitality ☐	Skin ☐	Bones ☐
Spacy ☐	Loving ☐	Joyful ☐	Balanced ☐	Strong ☐
Grief ☐	Greed ☐	Anger ☐	Lustful ☐	Fearful ☐

Fig. 1

3 Diagnosis

Diagnosis, like taking a case history, is an ongoing process that is important in every session that you give. To diagnose properly you need to re-evaluate the client's condition at the beginning of each session and also during actual treatment. It is possible to separate diagnosis into two categories, physical and energetic. Dr. Stone wrote extensively concerning physical diagnosis and so we will begin our look at the diagnostic process here.

Physical diagnostic procedures are based upon the convenience of the patient, that is to say, they should all be done at the beginning of the session before the actual bodywork begins, and as far as possible should not involve the client having to get on and off the table a number of times. The first diagnostic procedure is done using the gravity board to ascertain the way in which the client organises their physical structure in relation to gravity. This subject is dealt with in depth in the chapter on structural balancing later in this book. The second diagnostic procedure is taking the client's blood pressure. This is most conveniently done with the client sitting on the bodywork table. It should be taken on both sides of the body because the information so gained can be very useful in relation to balancing of the autonomic nervous system using perineal and coccygeal treatments. Remember that even though a client's blood pressure may register high, this is no reason to suppose that it is so at other times. There are many factors that can influence the blood pressure at the beginning of a treatment, not the least being nervous anticipation. The pulse rate may also be taken at this time. The radial pulse should be taken at both sides, as should the pulse at the carotid artery. Currently there are available automated sphagmanometers that register both blood pressure and pulse simultaneously, some even work by checking the blood pressure at the fingers which is infinitely more useful in that the blood pressure and pulse rate can be monitored throughout the session. When checking the pulse rate manually, do it quickly with a light touch as it is quite easy to create a false reading because excessive finger pressure influences it very quickly. The pulse can also be taken at other places on the body, which allows you to build up a picture of the overall distribution of life energy to the various areas of the body.

The third procedure is done with the client lying on the bodywork table, and it is to ascertain the short leg side. The short leg side indicates the side of the body on which there is an overall contraction of the electromagnetic currents of energy. It is basically caused by unequal muscle tension in the pelvis, and is a partial indicator of sacral positioning. It can be caused by physical injury or by a functional imbalance in the five elements.

The fourth procedure is to check the respiratory functioning. This is most easily done by placing your hands in different positions on the client's ribcage and checking the mobility of the different areas, as the client breathes both normally and when encouraged to breathe deeply. After doing this check the respiratory rate, the number of breaths that they take per minute. This gives you the overall picture of the functioning of the sympathetic nervous system. It tells you how much oxygen and prana the client is drawing from the atmosphere. You can correlate the number of breaths per minute to the pulse rate. A good balance is four heartbeats to every one breath. Should the respiratory rate be very slow and the pulse fast, then you could interpret this as indicating that whilst the circulation of energy may be good the actual quantity may be far less than is necessary for adequate functioning of the body.

Dr. Stone liked to check the nasal passages to see whether they were sufficiently open to allow a free flow of breath and prana. He also recommended using gold and silver dilators to open the passages. This is a technique that was developed at the turn of the century and works on the sympathetic reflex areas in the Shneiderian membrane of the nasal cavity. However, this technique is far beyond the scope of this book. You can effect a dilation of the nasal passages by doing deep breathing exercises using the alternate nostril breathing techniques of the yogic science of pranayama. It is important to encourage nasal breathing as it has a number of distinct advantages over mouth breathing. As the air passes through the nostrils it is cleaned and filtered by the hairs in the nose as well as being heated to a level that will not harm the sensitive internal membranes of the throat and lungs. The prana in the breath is absorbed directly into the brain via the nasal membranes and sinuses where it activates the cerebral cortex and the caduceus currents of energy.

The next thing to look at is exactly how the client's body is lying on the table. Look for any kind of angular distortions in the way that it is lying. For example you may find that the head

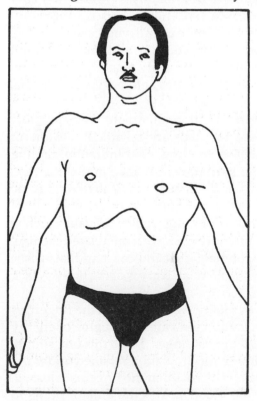

Fig. 2

19

and the torso seem balanced and symmetrically aligned, but that from the diaphragm area the body seems to veer off to the right or left (Fig. 2). It is possible that a client may show a number of angular distortions so that they are lying in a zig-zag fashion on the table. These angular distortions nearly always occur at the different chakra levels and are indicative of disturbances at the point where the distortion occurs. These distortions are indicative of imbalances in the flow of life energy in the body. They are not structural distortions because as the body is lying on the table gravity is no longer acting on it to the extent that it does when standing. What you see as the client is lying on the table is the way the flow of life energy directly affects the muscle structure and bodily alignment. When off gravity the position that the physical body adopts is a direct reflection of the inner flow of life energy without any secondary adaptations to gravity. This is because, as Dr. Stone pointed out, the life energy and the five elements are beyond the influence of gravity. Ideally this kind of body and energy reading would best be done with the client suspended in water. Unfortunately, this is not practical in the average treatment room! When reading the body in this way always look from the top of the table down the client's body and from the bottom of the table up, as it is sometimes easier to see distortions from one angle rather than another. What you are seeing is, in a sense, the client's inner relationships, how they feel about themselves, the dynamics of their self image and character structure. Unlike some therapies where it is recommended that the client is positioned symmetrically on the table, to do so in a polarity session is to lose out on the opportunity to gather a great deal more information towards your overall diagnosis.

It is also useful to check for hot and cold areas on the client's body. This is done by using the hands to pick up actual differences in the surface temperature. You are using your hands to detect problems with circulation, which is indicated predominantly by warm and cool areas. The hot areas are indicative of inflammation and excessive energy. Very cold areas are indicative of chronic energy blocks. Whilst this technique is quite useful, you have to be able to make some kind of differentiation between the terms warm, cool, hot and cold in relation to each client individually. It is important that the room is uniformly heated and that the client has been undressed and lying still for some five to ten minutes before trying to use this kind of diagnosis.

The final aspect of physical diagnosis is looking at the alignment and possible disfigurement of the fingers and toes. The finger and toe nails are reliable indicators of energetic disturbances, in as much as dryness, brittleness, splitting, discolouration, ridging of any particular finger or toe can be related to some kind of disturbance in the element, chakra and organs represented by it. As disturbances of the feet are indicative of chronic conditions and the hands of acute conditions, any severe disfiguration in the finger nails shows a chronic or dormant condition that is now becoming active. Usually such a disturbance in the finger nail will be matched by a similar problem with the related toe nail. The alignment of the fingers and toes is another useful diagnostic indicator, in that twists, bends and overlapping are also indicative of problems in the related areas of the body. A lack of mobility in any of the joints is another important factor.

Another useful diagnostic indicator is the amount of retained circulation in the fingertips when they are squeezed. The amount of retained circulation indicates the degree of energy flowing in any of the corresponding areas represented by that finger. To do this one simply squeezes the sides of the tip of the finger to see the amount of circulation retained under the nail. It is also useful to study the rate at which the blood returns when the finger is released. Check all the fingers and compare. Remember that the blood carries the bulk of prana in circulation in the body, so all the diagnosis based on blood flow is a direct indicator of energy flow. You can also sense differences in the circulation by squeezing the fingertips quickly and gently and comparing the elasticity and fullness of the tissue.

The bridge between purely physical diagnosis and purely energetic is the art of Ayurvedic pulse diagnosis. The blood is, as I said, the main carrier of the life energy. It is made up of three principles: the airy principle, which relates physically to the oxygen within the blood and energetically is the prana; the fire principle, which is the heat within the blood stream; and the water principle, which is the basic fluidic nature of blood. The pulse beat depends on these three principles for its rhythm and quality. In Ayurvedic pulse diagnosis the pulse is taken with the tips of the air, fire and water fingers. The information obtained relates physically to the pumping of the heart, the elasticity of the arteries and capillary pressure, and energetically to the three principles or, to use the Ayurvedic term, the three Doshas. The Doshas, which should not be confused with the five elements although they are related, are Vayu (air), Pitha (fire) and Kapha (water). The Doshas are the Ayurvedic term for the three forces that are active in any disease state or physical disharmony. They are perhaps most easily understood by the terms 'dry problems', 'hot problems', and 'watery problems', so any physical problem can be characterised by being caused by either too much or too little air, heat or water within the body. In Polarity terms the three Doshas could perhaps be understood as being related to the terms positive, neutral and negative. In which case, the air dosha would be the neutral phase of movement of energy, the fire dosha would be related to the positive phase of energy movement, and the water dosha to the negative phase. The Doshas are related to the five elements in the following way: the air dosha is a combination of the ether and air elements; the fire dosha is either the fire element alone or sometimes in combination with the water element (different schools of Ayurvedic medicine disagree on this); and the water dosha is a combination of the water and earth elements.

The particular qualities of the doshas could be summarized briefly as follows:

VAYU (Air) is the moving force of the living body and without it the other two doshas could not move. It is concerned with physical and mental processes which are dynamic in nature; sight, speech, hearing, etc., and perceptions in all physical and psychic manifestations. It sets and keeps in motion all other forces which are incapable of moving on their own. Vayu governs enthusiasm, respiration, motor activities (mental and physical). It regulates the autonomic nervous system. It manifests itself in any inflammatory state as pain. No pain is possible without Vayu. Vayu is light, cold, dry, mobile and piercing.

PITHA (Fire) is to heat, to burn or warm up. It is concerned with physical and mental processes which are balancing and transformative in nature; hunger, cheerfulness, intelligence, ideas, digestion, thirst. The function of Pitha is to regulate and maintain oxidation and supply heat as well as maintain thermal balance within the body.

KAPHA (Water) is the equivalent of cold in the body. It embraces and holds things together. It modifies and checks Pitha. It lubricates the body, especially the joints and skin. Kapha supports tissue growth. It produces courage, forbearance and vitality. Kapha is conserving and stabilizing in its effect.

As you can see, there is a definite relationship between the doshas and the elements, and from my own personal study of Ayurvedic medicine it seems to me that the three principles or doshas were conceptualised because Ayurvedic doctors found that the five element theory was too complicated when trying to devise appropriate therapeutic strategies.

To take the pulse you use the air, fire and water fingers of your right hand. When taking the pulse of a male client you take it at his right wrist, and of a lady client at her left wrist. The client's pulse is taken in such a way that your air finger is always the finger nearest to the base of the thumb. Its exact position is two finger-widths below the root of the thumb. The pulse is taken with the client sitting down. The client's arm is bent slantingly upwards, supported at the elbow by your free hand (Fig. 3). Their hand should be held so that the fingers point upwards as you take the pulse.

Do not try to take a client's pulse if they have just had a bath, shower, or meal, or if they have been exercising. Nor should they be hungry or thirsty. Basically, they need to be calm both mentally and physically.

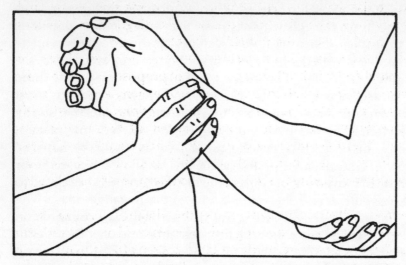

Fig. 3

Once you can feel the pulse you need to get a sense of what is happening under all three of your fingers. You are sensing the activity over quite a long section of the radial pulse. In Ayurvedic medicine there are considered to be some six hundred different pulse qualities. We are just going to look at a few of the main variations. The pulsation that you feel under the air finger relates to Vayu, under the fire finger relates to Pitha and under the water finger relates to Kapha. Firstly, it is always a good idea to define what that rarest of animals — a normal pulse beat — feels like. It is a pulse that can be felt under all three fingers with the sensation under each finger being slow, light and forceful. You should also be able to exert moderate pressure on the pulse without it being obliterated. It can only exist when all the three doshas are in harmony. Looking at the doshas individually the pulses related to them are:

Vayu a fast pulse, which feels as if it moves in curves like a snake.
Pitha a jumpy pulse. Its movement is like that of a frog or sparrow.
Kapha a slow pulse. Its movement is like that of a swan or peacock.

When sensing the pulse through your fingertips the first thing to ascertain is where you feel it. If it impinges mainly on your air finger then Vayu is out of balance, on your fire finger then Pitha is out of balance or on your water finger then Kapha is out of balance. If the pulse feels as though it is between the air and fire fingers, then both Vayu and Pitha are disturbed, and between your fire and water fingers then Pitha and Kapha are disturbed. If the pulse seems to come between all three fingers then all the doshas are out of balance. If you feel the pulse at all three fingertips but more strongly at one than the others, then the dosha corresponding to the finger where the pulse is strongest is disturbed. Having decided where you are feeling the pulse look to its quality. Is it fast, slow, or jumpy? Or to use the animal symbology, is it moving like a snake, a swan or a frog? If it at first seems fast and snakelike, then becomes jumpy or froglike and finally moves slowly like a swan, then the doshas are functioning in a regular fashion and this indicates an excellent prognosis in terms of the client making a full recovery. When all three doshas are disturbed the pulse will seem to be fast, slow and jumpy all at once. When the pulse moves alternately like a snake and then a frog, both Vayu and Pitha are disturbed. If it moves like a snake and then a swan, Vayu and Kapha are disturbed, and should it move like a frog and then a swan both Pitha and Kapha are in trouble.

The technique as outlined above is, I hope, clear and simple enough for anyone to learn the fundamentals of Ayurvedic pulse diagnosis. The only way to become skilful is through constant practise. Learning any of the oriental techniques of pulse diagnosis is a lifelong process, but the usefulness of the skill more than justifies the effort.

The other form of diagnosis which I also see as a bridge between the physical and the purely energetic procedures is foot and hand reflexology. I do not propose to go into these techniques in detail as they have been dealt with in great depth in the many excellent books available on the subject. However, a couple of points seem worth mentioning. Occasionally there are so many sore areas on a client's foot as to make you think that all their energy flows and related organs are disturbed. This phenomena is, in my experience, usually caused by a severe water element imbalance, very often in the pelvis. In this situation the hands will normally give a clearer picture. When checking the reflexes always flex the feet, as this helps to bring the reflexes to the surface.

Energetic diagnosis, sometimes called clairvoyant or psychic diagnosis, is the direct sensing of the state of a client's energy field by hearing, touch or vision. There is no 'sixth sense' involved in this process. It is done by developing an acute degree of sensitivity in one or more of the aforementioned senses. The most commonly developed channels for the information to be obtained through are sight and touch, though it is possible to 'hear' the energy, particularly by people with highly developed musical 'ears'. Energy is, after all, vibration just as is sound. My own particular skills are in sensing energy by touch and vision, so techniques that use these two senses are the ones I shall look at in detail.

Before looking at these techniques it is important to note that there is another technique that can be used to diagnose a client's condition, and this is by the use of a pendulum. A pendulum is simply a small, heavy weight made of either wood, metal or crystal that is attached to a piece of string or a chain that is about six to eight inches long. Pendulum diagnosis can be done even before you see a client, which is worth doing from the point of view of not making the client think that you are a bit strange, and also as a way of checking the accuracy of your 'dowsing' (to use the correct term). After using a pendulum for a period of time and becoming proficient in its usage, you often find that you no longer need it because you know where the problems are immediately at a conscious level. Dowsing is a way of accessing your own sub-conscious mind. It is also a way of familiarising yourself with the fact that you have a sub-conscious mind, an aspect of your consciousness which is intimately aware of life energy as it is the medium with which it controls the functioning of the body. It is through our sub-conscious mind and the fact that it can easily access information from the sub-conscious mind of the client, perhaps through the existence of the collective unconscious as well as some properties that are inherent in life energy, that we are able to diagnose the state of their energy. Using the pendulum is a way of training your sub-conscious mind in the particular language of energy that is used in polarity therapy until it can present it directly to your conscious awareness.

23

Learning to use the pendulum is very easy. All you need to do is calibrate it and then decide on the kind of questions you want to ask. To calibrate a pendulum is to clarify the kind of movement that it makes to indicate a 'yes' answer, and the movement that indicates a 'no' answer. When using the pendulum I have found it best if you support the elbow. Set the pendulum swinging very gently in a backwards and forwards oscillation (towards you and away from you) with a range of about one to two inches. Now ask the question either out loud or in your mind 'is my name . . .' using your full name. This is a question which must get an affirmative response, so the way in which the pendulum moves in relation to this question is its 'yes' answer, which may be the same back and forth movement you began with or a different one. Once again set the pendulum swinging very gently. Now ask a question the answer to which you know is going to be 'no', for example 'am I . . . years old' using a figure that is definitely wrong. The direction of movement you get in response to this question is your 'no' answer. Commonly people find that a 'yes' answer is some kind of circular swing and a 'no' answer a side to side or back and forth movement, or sometimes 'yes' is a clockwise circle and 'no' an anticlockwise circle. There really are no set rules. Initially it is best to check the calibration of the pendulum each time you use it until a set pattern is established. This usually only takes a short while but for the sake of accuracy it is worth doing at first.

The questions you ask in relation to a client's energy are almost limitless. You can ask about the functioning in the five elements, the activity of the chakras, the nervous system balance, check for blockages in the individual current lines, and so on. Always make sure that you understand the subject area that you are dowsing. In other words, if you do not understand the five element theory then do not ask questions about the balance of the elements, as the answers from the pendulum are not likely to be accurate. Remember it only reflects the understanding that your sub-conscious mind has of the language you are using, and if you do not understand elemental theory because you have not studied and comprehended it, how can you expect your sub-conscious to give you meaningful accurate answers. It is worth noting that using a pendulum in the manner I have outlined above is by no means the only way it can be used, any good book on dowsing will offer you many other possibilities.

What is often referred to as hand scanning is one of the simplest ways of feeling imbalances in the client's energy field. Remember that the energy field or aura extends way beyond the boundaries of the physical body. The aura itself is composed of many interpenetrating layers of energy, all vibrating at different frequencies. The layer of the aura that we are often most interested in is the so-called 'health aura', or sometimes the etheric double, which is the particular vibrations of energy that radiate from the core of the energy field to no more than one-half to one inch beyond the surface of the body. To scan this layer of the aura simply run your open palm slowly all over the surface of the body approximately one inch above it. What you are looking for are *changes* in sensation in the palm of your hand. There is no specific quality of sensation that you should experience. What you want to feel are the differences between the various areas you are scanning. The kind of sensations that you might experience are predominantly a mixture of heat, cold, tingling, vibration, pain, pulsation or pressure. The actual sensation that you get when sensing energy is going to be unique to you. This is not a skill that comes quickly, but it certainly is one that is worth cultivating. Feeling disturbances in a client's energy field is only the first step of this particular kind of psychic diagnosis. The ability to interpret the sensations that you experience, what they actually mean, is something that could take you many years of practice to achieve with any degree of clarity. There are many books that purport to define the meanings of the various sensations that you can experience whilst hand scanning. However, because everyone's experience is subtly different, there is really no reason to suppose that the information contained in books of this kind is going to be useful to you.

It is important when hand scanning to move your hands slowly over the body, because the sensations that you experience are very subtle. If you move your hand too quickly you will not give yourself time to absorb the various impressions. It is almost as if there is a time lag between your sense of touch picking up some variation and your conscious recognition of it. Having said that you should do the technique slowly, if you do it too slowly you will actually begin to manipulate the flow of energy in that particular area just as if you were giving a treatment. If there is a rule when practising hand scanning it is 'first impressions count'. Re-checking any particular area more than once will also affect the energy there. You can practise this technique on yourself, which can be particularly useful in learning to interpret what you are feeling, especially if you have some specific problem areas that are easy for you to reach and scan with your palm. Some people find that one of their hands is more sensitive than the other when doing this kind of diagnosis. Quite often it is the left hand, but again it is a personal preference. Scanning the physical or health aura tells you a great deal about the physiological functioning of the body. It is also possible to scan the aura further from the body than the boundaries of the health aura, out into the layers of the aura that correlate with the different levels of the mind.

Scanning the auric shell between one to ten inches off the body corresponds to the sub-conscious mind and emotions. It is sometimes called the astral area of the aura. Scanning from ten inches to two feet off the body corresponds to the conscious mind and thoughts, and from two feet off the body to the boundaries of the aura (which varies) relates to the super-conscious mind and soul. Checking all of the aura from the physical to the super-conscious area can reveal much concerning an energy disturbance that you detect at the physical level, as should there be a disturbance further off the body in the same area you can deduce whether the problem has emotional, mental or spiritual factors involved. As some clients can find it rather strange if you scan the outer layers of the aura, not being used to seeing someone floating their hands some way off their body, I usually ask them to relax and close their eyes for a few moments whilst I do it. I personally find it something of a distraction watching the bemused expression on their face if they keep their eyes open!

What I call deep scanning is a variation of hand scanning. It involves projecting the energy from your palm down into the body to ascertain exactly where the source of the energy imbalance that is manifesting at the surface of the body actually is. The ability to detect the actual source of any particular energy disturbance can make your release work much more specific and effective. If you remember that all the different frequencies of life energy begin at the core and radiate outward, it is obvious that many of the disturbances that you detect in the physical aura will have their roots much deeper in the body's energy fields. The Hermetic concept of 'as within, so without' also relates to this phenomena. The actual technique is to place your hand on the surface of the body and project your energy like a beam which will be reflected back to you, the source, when it meets an obstacle. A radar or sonar beam acts in just this fashion when it meets an object. The effectiveness of this technique depends upon your awareness. Remember that your intention moves your energy. What you are looking for is an awareness of a resistance or a complete blockage to the free movement of your energy as you project it into the body. With practice it is possible to determine quite precisely the exact depth and size of any energy blockage in the client's energy field. Not all disturbances in the physical aura will be coming from a deeper level. When you place your hand on the body to do deep scanning and you have a feeling that your energy and awareness can not penetrate beneath the surface, that they are scattered instantly, then you could expect that you were picking up tension or armouring in the superficial muscles in that area. When you come to trying to release the blockage that you have discovered, by whatever technique that you think appropriate, the perception that you have of its actual depth and position will enormously enhance the clarity of your intention, which in turn will ensure a full clearance of the energy field.

After working with energetic diagnostic techniques for some length of time and having become very familiar with the life energy by giving many sessions, you will probably find that you will begin to 'see' the energy. A visual as opposed to kinesthetic perception of the life energy is not necessarily more accurate, but it is certainly faster. It is true to say that some people are far more adept at feeling the aura than they ever could be at seeing it. Indeed I would say that everybody can learn to feel energy but not everyone can learn to see it. To be able to see something which is not physical requires the ability to let go of your normal everyday visual models of reality. For some people this is impossible, because it would mean a loss of psychological stability. Initially you will see the energy with your peripheral vision, out of the corner of your eye, so to speak. Do not try to chase or force the phenomena, just notice it when it happens and accept that it will probably become more frequent. There are various systems of eye exercises that are designed to facilitate your visual perception of the aura, and certainly they work for some people. To be able to see it really clearly requires you to be able to enter what is basically an altered state of consciousness, so meditation practice and experience with hypnotic states can be beneficial in helping to expand your world view to encompass the ability to see the energy that is the essence of life.

Ultimately, by continuing to practise all these diagnostic techniques you will in all probability reach a point where your sub-conscious mind has assimilated them so well that you will simply 'know' what the sources of a client's energy imbalances are without actually performing any of the diagnostic procedures outlined above. At this point you will have transcended technique and have moved into artistry.

4 Second Thoughts

The practice of Polarity Therapy lies in a grey area between Body-Orientated Psychotherapy and Alternative Medicine, the particular emphasis, be it psychotherapy or alternative medicine, being at the discretion of the individual practitioner. I believe that Polarity Therapy as taught and practised by Dr. Stone was a powerful form of drugless healing, and so would come under the generic title of Alternative Medicine. The psychotherapeutic approach is a more recent development created by students who already had a background either in counselling or in the various body-orientated forms of psychotherapy such as Reichian Therapy or Bioenergetics. It will therefore be of some interest to look at the major current models of psychotherapeutic practice so as to see perhaps where your own approach lies.

Having a clear sense of the model that you are using with any particular client will give a better foundation upon which both you and your client can judge the effectiveness of the work and allow the contract between you to be unambiguous. It is also important to remember that you do have to limit yourself to using just one model in your practice. I have often found myself working for a few months as an Alternative Medical practitioner, followed by a few months as a psychotherapist and so on. Indeed the model that you use often seems to be dictated by the universal law of attraction. If you are going through a period of emotional readjustment then those are the kind of clients you will attract and you will be doing psychotherapy, or if you are experiencing aches and pains or have recently injured yourself you will attract clients who need drugless healing. It all depends on exactly where your consciousness is at any particular time.

All current systems of psychotherapy have a therapeutic model, that is an overall concept of the way the particular system being used functions. Currently the two major models in usage are content and process based therapy. These approaches can then be either strategic or client centred. The content model of psychotherapy is based upon the concept that for a resolution of the client's problems it is necessary for them to become consciously aware of the roots, at the sub-conscious level, of the reasons for their particular problem; in essence the belief being that if we know why we are doing or experiencing something that is a problem, it will change. It could also be called an insight model, in that it relies on insight into the nature and causes of a particular problem to provide a stimulus to change. The main content question is 'why?'. The major problem with doing purely content-based therapy in this day and age is that people are fundamentally far more sophisticated in their understanding of psychological patterns, and unless the roots of their problems lie in an area with which they have no familiarity the insight gained will not have any appreciable impact on their problem. Freudian Psychoanalysis is the classic example of a therapy that uses a content model. In the time period in which it was developed, showing clients that the roots of their problems lay in the oedipal situation had an enormous psychological impact simply because it was not an area of human relationships that anyone had really previously looked at in any depth. I believe that there is in all of us a desire to know why something is the way it is. It is the basic drive behind all scientific discovery in every field, the essential curiosity of the human being without which we would still be living in caves.

The process model is based upon the concept that it is not why we do something, but the process or the steps that cause a particular problem that are significant. An understanding of how we go about creating a particular problem is the main aim of process-orientated therapy. Once we understand how we create a particular problem we can then interfere consciously in the process or steps we would normally take and create a new outcome for ourselves. Process therapy focuses a great deal of attention on the flow of feelings in the mind-body continuum. It looks at such things as body movement, posture, voice tone, etc., as indicative of the feeling stream in relation to the content of any particular experience. Awareness practices often form a large part of process-orientated therapy, learning to become aware of tension patterns in the body, discovering how you feel about your body, and so on. Process questions are 'how, when, where, what?'. Gestalt therapy and Neuro-Linguistic Programming are examples of therapeutic systems that largely use the process model.

Apart from the therapeutic model there is what I call the therapeutic approach. It is the basic structure of the relationship between therapist and client. There are two main approaches at this time, 'strategic' and 'client centered'. The strategic approach to therapy, be it based on the content or process model, occurs when the therapeutic techniques are decided by the therapist without consultation with the client. In the strategic approach the therapist's role is that of strategist who plans a campaign of action down to the finest details, who evaluates the effects of the actions taken, modifies any plans according to the responses and evaluates the outcome himself. Although the client will usually specify some kind of desired outcome during the initial consultation, if they do not the therapist will create a series of therapeutic changes based on his own evaluation of the client's needs. The strategic approach may well take a client far beyond any original request for a particular outcome. This sometimes happens because the strategy used to effect a particular outcome may have far greater ramifications than implied in the original request, and the techniques used create change at such a fundamental level that much more is derived from the therapy than the client originally intended. In the strategic approach the therapist takes full responsibility for the influence he exerts on the client. Eriksonian hypnotherapy is an example of strategic therapy.

The client-centred model is based upon the therapist initiating no therapeutic interventions until the client is able to articulate their needs. The idea being that if a client has a problem but does not know what to do about it, then the therapist should involve them fully in the decision making process by reflecting back their comments in a passive way until sufficient clarity develops in the mind of the client as to what they actually want out of the therapy. This is an ongoing element in the therapy, the client specifying the therapeutic outcome and being fully involved in the therapy, making new choices in full consultation with the therapist as the work progresses. There is an avoidance of any sense of manipulation of the client by the therapist as being 'dis-empowering', as taking away their sense of being in control of their lives. In the client-centered approach the responsibility for

28

the nature of the work lies with the client. Humanistic psychology tends to use the client-centred model.

To a great extent any but the most ardent purists within any particular system of psychotherapy will probably use more than one model in their practice. Nearly all practitioners of process-orientated therapy will make some interpretations at various points in their work. Practitioners of content-orientated therapy will also focus on process periodically. However, it would be rare to find a therapist who uses both the client-centred approach and the strategic approach. Most practitioners will opt for one of the approaches and stay with that throughout their working life as a therapist.

Most systems of psychotherapy have a particular conceptual model of the 'healthy human being'. The definitions of such a person range from someone who is free of all neurosis, to a person capable of a full orgasm, to someone who is self actualising. Any therapy is to a great extent orientated, whatever its model, to turning the client into its own vision of a healthy person. The existence of such models of a perfect human being means that whatever the desired outcome of the therapy as specified by the client, the course of the therapy must be subordinated to the therapist actualising within the client the model of perfect human functioning that they ascribe to. For instance, a client comes to a therapist whose model of perfect functioning is a person capable of a full orgasm. The client's specific desire is to overcome certain anxieties in relation to their working life, perhaps their ability to deal with authority figures. The only way that the therapist can achieve this is by seeking to make the client able to express their concept of perfect functioning, because if they can achieve this then all the client's problems will disappear. Admittedly this is a simplistic interpretation of what is in fact an exceedingly complex process, but in essence it is a valid statement. It is as well to know the kind of concept of a healthy human being that a therapist subscribes to before undergoing any therapeutic work with them. These models often contain a number of inbuilt limitations that you may not wish to take on board.

As a polarity therapist, what do you feel is your concept of a healthy human being? What was the model expressed during your training? In some training courses the model is not taught openly but has to be inferred from many different statements concerning human behavioural patterns. It is always possible to reduce the model offered, whether openly or covertly, no matter how seemingly complicated, to a few simple statements or even a single phrase. The polarity concept of a healthy individual according to Dr. Stone is a person with abundant free flowing energy and who has a sense of connection with the source of all life, and to this I would add, who also has the ability to change easily.

The therapeutic contract, like any contract, is an agreement between two parties concerning some form of business arrangement. If you practise polarity therapy as a system of alternative medicine then the contract that you enter into with the client will be fairly simple. It will be to the effect that you as a therapist undertake to restore, as far as is possible, normal functioning in their body as quickly as is feasible, and that they undertake to come for a specified number of sessions or until the problem is resolved, and further that they will pay for this service. The important factor here is that it would be unwise, from the practitioner's point of view, to make any categoric statement to the effect that the client will definitely get better. It is as well to remember that in England it is against the law to make claims of possessing an ability to cure certain diseases. Any false or exaggerated claim on the part of the practitioner is going to undermine the relevance of any contract, if not totally invalidating it.

If you practise polarity therapy as a form of body and energy based psychotherapy then the contract between you and your client needs to cover a broader spectrum of issues. The practitioner's side of the contract needs to cover such details as cost, the number of sessions, the point at which some form of mutual review of therapeutic progress is undertaken, the kind of therapy that is offered, an explanation of the possible effects of the therapy and the confidentiality of personal information. It should also specify any ground rules to be followed during the actual session; for example, if you are doing a lot of counselling, is the client allowed to smoke? If you use some form of cathartic emotional release work, is violence against you prohibited or would it be permissible for the client to physically wrestle with you? Do you offer telephone support to the client outside of normal business hours? The client's side of the contract covers such issues as payment on time, punctuality, an agreement to offer, as far as is possible, information both honestly and openly, and that if any issues arise over which they are in any way unsure, they will clarify them with the practitioner. Actually going for therapy implies, at least at some level, a willingness on behalf of the client to change, which, if you like, is part of the implicit unspoken aspects of the contract.

My own opinion of the fundamental model on which polarity therapy is based is that it is a process model. Working with the life energy is working with the essential ground of being, the dance of life. It is impossible to talk about the flow of life energy in the body in terms of 'why'. The energy just 'is'. I use a strategic approach in the polarity work that I do. I practise polarity both as alternative medicine and psychotherapy. With some clients I find the work shifts from alternative medicine to psychotherapy during treatment, thereby necessitating the negotiation of a new contract.

There is the possibility of another model of approach to polarity therapy which is not client-centred or strategic, in that it does not offer the client any specific outcomes. It is non-directive and is not even 'therapy' in the normal usage of the term, although the effects can certainly be therapeutic. I call this approach the 'attunement approach'. It seeks to attune the client to the existence of life energy and its flow in the body through the experience of the energy work. It is all about giving the client an experience in its purest form without any interpretation or explanations. It is polarity for personal growth in the sense of a growth in consciousness or knowingness of life, to know what it is to be 'alive'. It is trusting that the life energy has consciousness and wisdom, and that it will create the most appropriate changes in the client because the prana, the breath of life, is also the breath of the soul, and it is the soul that truly knows what we need and how we should be in this life. An attunement to the life energy is, when done properly, the creation of a channel of communication with your own soul. To practise polarity therapy in this way is to no longer be locked in a therapist/client relationship but to be joint adventurers in the exploration of the subtle realms.

The attunement approach involves a joining and resonance at the level of the soul, where two unique individuals, freed from the confines of matter, can soar and dance in the quest for the source of all life. It is the Taoist return to the source that is beyond death whilst still being fully involved in the process of life. This particular approach to polarity is best attempted upon a solid foundation of practical and theoretical knowledge of the system. It is not an excuse for ineptitude. The attunement approach is an approach that transcends any concept of therapy, and could perhaps be expressed in the form of a Taoist paradox stated as 'Therapy, Non-Therapy', or that one learns and practises therapy so that you do not have to do it. It is an approach that holds to the idea that the most effective therapeutic changes come out of a profound relationship between the people involved.

5   The Five Elements

One of the most fundamental aspects of Polarity Therapy is an understanding of the five element theory. Having studied Dr. Stone's books and many books on Ayurvedic medicine, as well as consulting with various people who were supposed to understand the theory, I found myself getting more and more confused. The main source of my confusion was a statement in Dr. Stone's writings to the effect that the five elements were like the plates in a battery which were energised by the life energy or prana. This seemed to indicate that he saw the five elements as energised substances, and yet I have also seen the theory stated that the five elements are fundamentally just five different qualities of energy in movement. Dr. Stone also wrote at various times of the five elements as matter and at other times as energy. My confusion only began to clear when I realised that in Ayurvedic medicine there are the five elements which are different vibrations of life energy, and the five tanmatras (five fundamental atoms) which have the same names as the five elemental energies. There is a chart in Dr. Stone's writings called the Pentamarius combination of the elements (discussed later in this chapter), which is actually the classification of the make-up of the five tanmatras and not, as I originally thought, the five elemental energies. In point of fact you cannot separate the five elements and the five tanmatras. The simplest way I can explain this relationship — and let me hasten to point out that is just my understanding — is that all matter is composed of different fundamental atoms, the five tanmatras, and that each of these atoms is energised by a specific vibratory rate of prana; for example, the earth or prithvi tanmatra is energised by the earth vibration of prana which is distributed throughout the body by the earth chakra. Note that the name for the earth elemental energy is also prithvi. The actual make-up of the earth tanmatra is one half pure earth and the other half equal quantities of the other four atoms, but its basic nature is earthy because that is the quality of life energy that infuses it. When these fundamental atoms become charged with the life energy, they attract each other through polarity and tend to have certain areas of the body where they congregate in great numbers, creating a particular oval field or area of activity, though all are present in varying quantities throughout the body.

With this understanding in mind we can now look at the manipulations in Polarity Therapy as having two different phases. The first, in which we work on the distribution of the elemental energies throughout the body by working on the chakras and the nervous system, and the second phase where we seek to repolarise the different fields of the body so that the energised atoms can attract each other and work harmoniously together. To give an example, suppose a client has a problem with their breathing which is obviously related to their air chakra and the air oval field, so your therapeutic work will be a combination of checking that the air chakra is functioning adequately and distributing its energy throughout the chest to the air tanmatras, and then by polarising the air oval field, ensuring that the re-energised air tanmatras are then attracting each other and working in harmony.

In a sense it is impossible to separate the concept of the five elements and the five tanmatras as they both function together, and we could say that all matter is energy anyway. I am not saying that the above model is anything other than a description of a subtle reality that is easy to grasp and work with. Your work must be based upon a clarity of mind that allows you to practise with confidence, even though it is not possible to define reality which is always greater than our ability to conceptualise accurately.

Dr. Stone pointed out that unless the five elements (the energised finer fundamental atoms) within our body are polarised appropriately, we cannot attract the finer essences of matter (the tanmatras) from our diet to replenish our energy fields and thereby maintain our structure. I have found that the model that I have just presented really helped to clarify what Dr. Stone meant when he talked about polarisation and de-polarisation, and how this differs from his discussion of the five rivers of energy. The terms polarisation and de-polarisation relate to the ability of the finer *substances* to attract their constituent components for balanced functioning. The 'one energy' which is modulated by the chakras is that which activates the finer essences of matter and gives them the ability to attract and repel.

The five different vibrations of prana flow throughout the whole of the body. They are created as a modulation or step down of the primary current of free prana in the atmosphere which we take in by breathing, and which is transferred by the sinuses to the brain. Once the prana is in the brain it is passed down the body via the caduceus currents. In the process of flowing down the body it is modulated at various power stations along the way, the chakras, so as to enable it to perform different functions in the body. The chakras are five different centres of energetic activity that occur down the length of the spinal column, where it is the action of our consciousness that transforms the prana into different vibrations. The chakras are centres of consciousness and energy. When the free prana comes in to the body it is undifferentiated, pure volitionless energy. The action of our consciousness at the chakra centres gives it a quality of volition or mindfulness. In simple terms it knows what it has to do. It is due to the fact that life energy is imbued with consciousness and because it flows in quite different channels from that of our ordinary nervous system that we have the possibility of a full and total perception of the structure of our body at the most subtle essence level of existence. A perception cultivated in many spiritual traditions as the true meaning of the phrase 'man know thyself'.

As our consciousness itself moves through phases of fear and negativity in response to inner self reflections about outer experience conveyed to it by the central nervous system, so the energy from the chakras can be imbued with certain negative or fearful qualities. When the modulated energy from a chakra carries a vibration of negativity with it, it does not polarise the fundamental atoms properly, so physical malfunctioning can often occur. It also creates the basis of the cellular memory. These energy based cellular memories are what is so often activated by a polarity treatment. What actually happens is that as the fresh energy is brought to an area where the atoms carry this kind of energy based memory, the old stagnant memory-laden energy is displaced and returns to the chakra that created it, and its content is then once more brought back in to conscious awareness.

As the chakras are the medium through which certain qualities of consciousness influence the body, it seems relevant to look at the particular qualities associated with each chakra. The throat chakra qualities, when the consciousness is in balance, are the feelings of reverence and bliss. The sense of actually being a soul. When the consciousness is out of balance then the feeling is one of grief, a loss of connection with the source of all life. At this chakra level the one life energy as manifested by God is changed or modulated the least from its original nature, which indicates that the state of consciousness related to this chakra is that quality of consciousness so sought after in the mystical experience of oneness with the universe, and which functions as spiritual aspiration. The particular quality of the energy is one of space.

The balanced qualities of consciousness at the heart or air chakra level are the soul qualities of love, compassion and imagination. The consciousness when disturbed manifests as hatred, desire or wanting things that you do not have, and chasing shadows. At this chakra level the modulation of the one life force functions as the need to relate to others. The particular quality of the energy is mobility.

The qualities of consciousness at the solar plexus or fire chakra are joy and enthusiasm. The sense of self and the body. The feelings at this level when the consciousness is unbalanced is anger and rage. At this level the modulation of the one life energy is at a point of balance and functions as the need to expand and grow to full self realisation. The quality of the energy is heat.

The qualities of consciousness at the sacral or water chakra level are courage, determination and fortitude, the sense of gender. When the consciousness is unbalanced it manifests as the feeling of greed, I have it but I want more. The modulation of the one life energy is functioning as racial drives which manifest as the protective instincts. The quality of the energy is smoothness.

The qualities of consciousness associated with the base or earth chakra are the sexual desires, when unbalanced consciousness at this level manifests as fear. The modulation of the one energy is ensuring the continuing function in the universe of the one life energy through the creation of new life by the sexual act. The quality of the energy is stability.

The five oval fields of the body are five cavities within the body where there are concentrations of various different kinds of activities. The five elements (or the five energised tanmatras) tend to congregate so that the fire element is in the head oval, the ether element in the throat oval, the air element is in the chest oval, the earth element in the abdominal oval and the water element in the pelvic oval (Fig. 4). All the elements are present throughout the body but these are the areas in which their *physical* functioning predominates. The water element position in this chart represents its major physical function as reproduction, the earth element position as digestion, the air element position as respiration, the ether element as speech, and the fire element position as vision and mental direction.

The five elements also have specific areas where they are most active as energy and consciousness. The air energy is most active in the head as constantly moving airy mind patterns. The ether energy is most active in the throat cavity as the underlying link between all the energy in the body, the communication channel or beam. The water energy in the chest as the emotional energy. The fire energy in the abdominal cavity as the source of the heat in the body. The earth energy in the pelvic cavity as the sexual energy (Fig. 4).

The Pentamarius combination of the elements is the elemental constitution of a number of different aspects of the human being.

The *ether* combinations are categorised as follows: Grief is the principle quality of ether, a feeling of nothingness. Desire is produced by a combination of air and ether. Anger is a

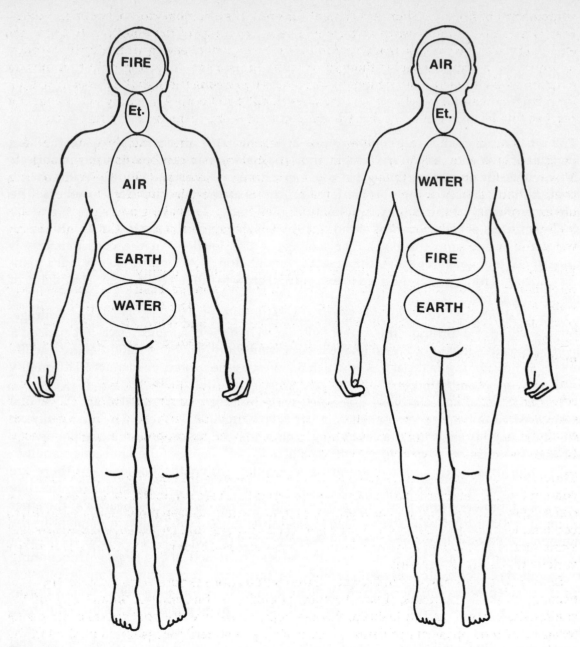

Fig. 4

combination of fire and ether. Attachment (or greed) is a combination of water and ether. Fear is a combination of earth and ether. The relationship of the emotions to the ether element is clear if we realise that an emotion is a movement of energy or feeling in the body to which we ascribe a specific thought or value judgement. A feeling only becomes an emotion when it reaches our conscious awareness by passing through the throat area, both for recognition and evaluation at a mental level, but also because it is only when a feeling reaches this level in the body that we can emote it, that is express it or bring it out.

The *air* combinations are as follows: Speed (mobility) is the principle quality of Air. Lengthening is a combination of ether and air. Shaking is a combination of fire and air. Movement (fizzing or bubbling) is a combination of water and air. Contraction is a combination of earth and air. The relationship of air to certain qualities of movement is obvious, one only has to study nature or your own body, the shaking and shivering of our bodies to warm up when cold (air/fire), and the white water effect as air stirs up and moves water, for example.

The *fire* combinations are as follows: Hunger is the main quality of fire. Sleep is a combination of ether and fire. Thirst is a combination of air and fire. Lustre is a combination of water and fire. Laziness is a combination of earth and fire. The fire combinations are all physiological drives, the need to eat, sleep, drink, have sex and relax. Air and fire are quite capable of drying out water, making you thirsty. Ether is capable of spacing out the fiery mental activity, making you sleep.

The *water* combinations are as follows: Semen is the main quality of water. Saliva is a combination of ether and water. Sweat is a combination of air and water. Urine is a combination of fire and water. Blood is a combination of earth and water. The water combinations are all bodily fluids. Saliva (or mucus) being produced in bodily cavities (ether). Sweat being produced by movement (air).

The *earth* combinations are as follows: Bones are the principle quality of earth. Hair is a combination of ether and earth. Skin is a combination of air and earth. Blood vessels are a combination of fire and earth. Flesh is a combination of water and earth. The earth combinations are all solid matter in the body. Skin is earth and air because it breathes and eliminates, flesh is water and earth because of its semi-solid sponge-like quality and all the various fluids that it contains.

Some of the reasoning behind certain of the combinations is not always clear but they will become clear if you think them through carefully — honestly! A knowledge of the combinations can be an invaluable tool when trying to discover the root causes in elemental terms of various physical problems. There is a nice treatment for insomnia implied in the combinations. Effective too!

You can balance any individual element by working on the appropriate oval field in the body using bi-polar contacts. To do this you have to imagine each field as a three-dimensional structure with a central point. To polarise any sore or blocked area in the field you make proportional contacts based on the distance of the blocked area to the central point. What this means is you imagine a line from a sore point through the centre of the field continuing on to an equidistant point on the other side. You then stimulate each point alternately until the blockage is cleared. For example, when working the fire oval in the head a sore point on the middle of the occipital base near the foramen magnum will have a corresponding release point on the middle of the forehead, approximately above the third eye area. As all contacts made following this rule are diagonal contacts, you are stimulating the deep caduceus energy currents in the body. This concept is illustrated in two-dimensional form in figure 5.

It is possible to balance any two elements by using bi-polar contacts, one on the area of function of one of the elements in question, and the other on the area of function of the other element. This concept can be utilised when dealing with imbalances in the physical aspect of elemental function or the energetic. For example, in the Tummy Rock you will see that it is a balancing of the Fire and Water Elements (the left-hand contact on the head representing the fire element in its physical area of manifestation, the right hand on the pelvis representing the water element in its area of physical manifestation). If you look at the technique and the contact areas from an energetic viewpoint it is a balancing of the Air and Earth elements (Air relating to the head and Earth relating to the pelvis).

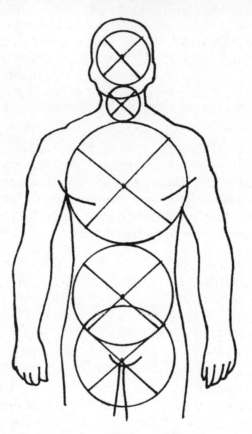

Fig. 5

Most polarity techniques that are done on the central vertical axis of the body with the hands separated by a distance of at least ten inches will be a balancing of two or more elements. A contact on the chest combined with one just below the diaphragm could be considered to be a balancing of the Air and Earth elements, if we look at the contact areas in terms of the physical manifestation of the elements, looked at energetically the same two contacts would be a balancing of Water (Chest) and Fire (the oval field beneath the diaphragm). This one technique could have a balancing effect on four elements at the same time. The coccyx treatment, in which the ganglion of impar is balanced against muscular tensions in the buttocks, could be said to be a balancing of Earth, Air, Fire, and Water. This is clear when you realise that the coccyx is the physical location of the earth chakra (earth), and is the location of the negative pole of the sympathetic nervous system, the ganglion of impar (fire). Looking at the buttocks we see that they are the physical motor pole of the water element. The buttock area is also a contact area for the para-sympathetic nervous system in that the sacral nerves are influenced (air), and in a general sense the treatment also affects the cerebrospinal impulses (air). Once again four elements are being balanced.

The only thing that will precisely define the effect of any treatment is where your mental intention lies; clarify that and your work will become specific to the balance between the particular elements that will be of most benefit to the client. Balancing any individual element is important, but we must remember that they do not exist in isolation, so learn to use the technique outlined above. Study the way that you work. What are you actually doing? Where is your intention?

It is also possible to balance two elements by working on their related reflex patterns. As an example: in the diaphragm releasing manipulation in which one hand is placed on the shoulder and the other hand is working out any tenderness in the buttocks, you are balancing the Air and Water Elements, the Air Element being represented in the shoulder contact (Air Element Triad: Shoulders, Kidneys, Ankles) and the Water Element represented in the buttock contact (Water Element Triad: Breasts, Genitals, Feet, the buttocks being the posterior motor positive pole of the genitals). You can also work reflex areas of one element to the oval field of the other to balance them both.

Dr. Stone wrote that any energy block is by definition, in its inception, a disturbance of the air element. The energy has stopped moving. The problem can be resolved quickly by working fire and water simultaneously. Working fire and water together will create a lot of air (or steam, to be exact) that will push through the blockage. However, this will not work if the blockage has become crystallised, as you would then be trying to resolve an earth element problem. Different elements would require stimulating and balancing. From this it is obvious that you should not just be considering balancing an element when it is disturbed by simply working on it and its reflex patterns in isolation, but be looking at the secondary effects of working two elements simultaneously as possibly being a far more effective route. A problem manifesting as a serious disturbance in one element may actually have its source in some low level disturbance in one or more of the others. If you were treating an acute fire problem, which of the following approaches would be best? To stimulate water and relate it to the fire patterns, as water controls fire; to stimulate earth in relation to fire, so that the fire is suffocated; to stimulate ether to space the fire out, so that it loses its concentrated power? What about cross-balancing earth and air, making stimulating contacts on the earth reflex patterns and satvic contacts on the air reflex patterns, thereby using earth to suffocate the fire, at the same time as you are calming and balancing the air that is fuelling the fire? What would be the most effective approach? Unfortunately there are no rules that will help you. You just have to follow your intuition for each individual client. Always be flexible in your approach and do not be afraid to change your tack in the middle of a treatment.

Having been a student for many years of both the western and eastern traditions of esoteric philosophy, and more recently of the oceanic cultures of the Pacific, I have yet to come across anything even remotely approaching a definitive system. All schools of thought have their good points and their weak points. I myself have worked with a number of other approaches to the energy balancing work apart from the five elements, from a mind energy model to a transpersonal approach that transcends concepts of dualism, to the four principle approach. All these approaches are valid and it is my feeling that our ultimate goal as healers is to transcend all the various models, which are in their very nature incomplete, to a direct knowingness of the fundamentals of life and energy.

The Four Principles

The Four Principles is an interesting way of looking at the human body and human behaviour. They are by name, the Thinking Principle, the Going Principle, the Doing Principle, and the Being Principle. Each principle relates to a kind of activity. Activities which are common to all of us at various times and to different degrees. They each relate to a specific area of the human body and to specific energy patterns. It is possible to characterise any of your clients by the balance of the four principles that they manifest. It is also easy to see which of the principles is being over or under used. Then use this understanding to clarify the kind of energy balancing techniques that would be most appropriate for them. It is important to realise that the balance of the four principles will vary over a period of time. They are not fixed in any way, nor are we seeking to create some kind of perfect balance between their usage by the client. What we want is that they have the ability to flow easily from expressing one principle into another.

THE THINKING PRINCIPLE

The Thinking Principle is simply the amount of thinking that a person does; the degree to which they use their conscious mind, their rationality. It is obviously true that some of us do more thinking than others and that we vary from day to day in the amount of rational analytical thinking that we indulge in. It is also true that some people do very little thinking; that they come from a much more visceral, emotional base. I am sure we have all come across the client who says they do not think; that they are too stupid, silly or childish to be able to think something through. This is rarely the case unless they have some form of serious abnormality of the brain. Everybody is capable of thinking. It would be impossible to survive without the ability to think things through, though it would certainly be true to say that some of us are more adept at it than others. Thinking is an ability that can be developed and sharpened by any of us if we so wish.

Physically, the Thinking Principle relates to the head area. Energetically, it relates to the fire chakra and the fire triad, and the posterior aspect of the umbilical spiral. As soon as a client indicates any kind of a problem with their head, from headaches to spots, look for some kind of an imbalance in their Thinking Principle. Explore their attitudes to their own thinking capabilities. Do they find themselves getting stuck with repetitive patterns of thoughts? Do they think they are stupid? Do they spend vast amounts of time in self reflection and self analysis? There are many other questions you could ask. Why not do a little exploration of your own Thinking Principle as a way of familiarising yourself with the concept?

THE GOING PRINCIPLE

The Going Principle is a person's ability to move, to get up and go. The ability to change position in life. It is linked to the Thinking Principle because the ability to move in life has ramifications beyond the mere physical action of moving the body. Movement is a motor activity that is in the first instance often initiated by the mind. However, it is also true that movement can be initiated by basic survival mechanisms. These in themselves have little or nothing to do with conscious thought processes. When looking at a client's Going Principle not only are you going to be investigating their physical mobility and strength, but also looking at their ability to change their life situations, i.e. relationships, occupation, etc. For any movement to occur there must be good contact with a stable base (the Earth) to push off from. Check the contact that their feet make with the ground. A stable inner centre of gravity is also an important requirement before one can initiate effective movement. Look at their self image. How strong and accurate is that?

Physically the Going Principle relates to the pelvis, legs, and feet. Energetically it relates to the Fire, Water, and Earth chakras, their associated astrological triads, and the posterior aspect of the umbilical spiral. If a client has any problems in the lower half of the body, from the pelvis down to the feet, then you are looking for an imbalance in the Going Principle. Even sexual problems are linked to problems in the Going Principle, but rather than tell you the connection see if you can think it out for yourself!

THE DOING PRINCIPLE

The Doing Principle is directly related to a person's motivation. Do they get things done in life? How good are they at achieving the things they want to do? Once again it is linked to both the Thinking Principle and the Going Principle, as any action is first a process of ideation, and then a movement towards the manifestation of the idea ('I am *going* to do it'), and finally the process of actually doing it. We all 'do' things or we try and achieve something through our efforts. Doing and effort are for most people fundamentally related. If you are going to do something then it will require a certain amount of effort. Unfortunately few people realise that the more effort they make, very often the less they actually achieve. The amount of effort a person puts into a project is related to their ability to maintain sufficient motivation to see it through to its completion. The more effort it takes the harder it is to stay motivated, whereas the more gracefully and economically they can apply their energy the easier it is to see something through to its completion. The Doing Principle is therefore both a person's ability to 'do' things and their ability to see their actions through to a satisfactory completion.

Physically the Doing Principle relates to the middle and upper back, neck, shoulders, arms and hands. Energetically it relates to the Ether, Air and Fire chakras, their associated astrological triads and the joints of the upper body. It also relates to the posterior aspect of the umbilical spiral. Does a client ever complete anything, do they use their energy efficiently, do they even begin a project or are they always going to do it but never quite begin to act? Negative answers to these questions all point to a disturbance of the doing principle.

THE BEING PRINCIPLE

The Being Principle is very simply a person's ability to 'be', it is a tranquil inner space in which there is no volitional activity, a space in which to experience the effects of your actions and as such it is the final phase of a movement that begins with the Thinking Principle. It is the point in any activity where a person absorbs and self reflects upon their emotional and physical movements within the world. It is also the point at which learning takes place. The balanced manifestation of the Being Principle allows the sense of completion to become a part of a person's life. In some sense when we are simply being we are in touch with our own personal experience of God. To be able to 'do' effectively one must be able to 'be', but there has to be a balance between these two principles. People who are compulsively doing things rarely ever experience any satisfaction in their doingness because they never take time to self reflect, and people who are always just being never experience the joy of creativity.

Physically the Being Principle relates to the abdomen and front of the chest. Energetically it relates to the anterior aspect of the umbilical spiral, the five-pointed star and the long straight line currents of energy. A client manifesting an imbalance in their Being Principle will often experience problems with their vitality. Ascertaining a client's attitude towards such things as rest and relaxation can tell you much about their relationship to their Being Principle. Do they use prayer or meditation in their daily life, and do they regularly take stock of their lives? Do they allow themselves the time to experience the glow of satisfaction that comes after a job well done?

It should be obvious that the Four Principles can be related to the Five Elements, and in fact an exploration of their possible inter-relationships can prove to be extremely illuminating.

6 Mind and Energy

'Mind is the finest substance of matter operating in three bodies as three fields of consciousness. The Causal body is the pattern field of the mind; here it is the ideal or superconscious or higher conscious mind; in the etheric or emotional field, mind operates through the senses. It is the normal conscious mind; in the gross physical body, mind governs all involuntary functions and repairs. It operates as the sub-conscious mind'.

In the above quote from Dr. Stone's writings he classifies mind as being triune in nature. He divides it into three levels, sub-conscious, conscious and higher conscious. What are the energy patterns that relate to each level of consciousness? Some might ask whether this is even a viable question. It is my belief that there are different energy patterns that relate directly to each level of mind. I believe that it would be true to say that perhaps seventy-five percent of the techniques that Dr . Stone developed work on the energy patterns relating to the sub-conscious mind; the realm of feelings and the force behind the repair and maintenance functions of the body. Specifically these energy patterns are the five bi-lateral long-line currents, the five lower chakras, the east-west currents and the caduceus currents. Any work on these energy patterns can be considered to be working with the client's sub-conscious mind.

It is the sub-conscious mind that supervises all the repair work in the body. It holds all the basic survival mechanisms, as well as being the storehouse of the memory. It is the sub-conscious mind that gives us the sensations of energy flow in the body, the feelings that eventually become emotions when they are linked to certain thoughts by the conscious mind. My concept of the sub-conscious mind is that it is a creature of habit. It likes patterns, particularly stable ones, and it is also remarkably stubborn. I see its basic function as the maintenance of patterns. It would be a very difficult life if we had to consciously maintain the physiological functioning of our body. Can you imagine what it would be like to have to consciously keep your heart beating; if every breath had to be conscious; if you had to direct the whole digestive process as well as attending to all the necessary repair work in the body? The sub-conscious does all these things for us. To do these tasks effectively it must store a vast number of patterns. These patterns contain extremely detailed information on the functioning of the body. The sub-conscious is constantly matching body function to these patterns, much like a computer system runs an executive programme to maintain its basic functioning capabilities.

The sub-conscious mind is also able to learn new patterns with remarkable ease. Patterns

41

that do not just relate to behavioural patterns or practical skills but that also relate to altered patterns of physiological functioning. This basic ability is one that we use all the time in our everyday lives. The classic example is learning to drive a car. This is an activity that has to be studied consciously with great attention to detail in its initial stages until we have learned the patterns of behaviour needed to do it effectively. These patterns are at a certain point then shifted to the sub-conscious mind, which stores them and enacts them whenever we require access to that particular skill, leaving our conscious mind free to attend to other matters. In the case of driving a car we all know when this has happened because suddenly we have sufficient free conscious attention to be able to hold a conversation and drive fluidly at the same time. The same process occurs as we grow up. We are taught certain patterns of behaviour by the adults around us which in the course of time become sub-conscious patterns that we use automatically. These kind of learned patterns form the basis of our character.

Once a pattern has been stored the sub-conscious mind will in general hold on to it indefinitely. Patterns which relate to physical functioning are normally held with greater tenacity than patterns which relate to behaviours, but as all patterns have survival value on some level this distinction is not always valid. The sub-conscious mind uses all the different patterns held within the memory as the blueprint for modulating the flow of energy and consciousness in the body. It is these patterns which determine the volume and direction of energy flow that underlie the physical and emotional structure of the body. In any trauma where distortion of the physical structure occurs the energy flow becomes distorted, which instantly shows up in the sub-conscious as a pattern disruption. This in turn sets in motion the basic survival mechanism, whereby the sub-conscious mind will begin to manipulate the energy until it again matches the appropriate pattern stored in the memory, so that healing at the physical level can take place.

In some case where the physical damage is too great or if there are other behavioural patterns of a conflicting nature being activated, then chronic unresolvable energetic imbalances will result and no physical healing will occur. For example, a client falls injuring their knee. In normal circumstances the sub-conscious will rebalance the energy and healing will begin, but if at this particular time in their personal life they are experiencing a definite lack of attention from their partner, and should they have stored a behavioural pattern to the effect that they receive a lot of attention when ill or incapacitated in some way, the net result is going to be that both patterns are going to be activated simultaneously and the sub-conscious is not going to be able to rebalance the energy due to the conflicting nature of each pattern. The need of the attention pattern in this case will override the basic healing pattern. The conflict will only resolve itself if the needs of the attention pattern become satisfied, which in turn will depend on the responses of the client's partner. This kind of resolution will not always occur, particularly if the relationship between the client and their partner was fundamentally damaged before the accident. The required increase in attention will not, in all probability, happen and the attention pattern will continue to block the healing. To resolve this kind of situation some form of outside therapeutic intervention is needed to help to de-activate the attention pattern.

All long-standing illness, disease and energetic imbalance can be thought of as a conflict of patterns in the sub-conscious mind. In this situation you are going to have to work diligently not only to get the energy unblocked and flowing freely, but to work simultaneously with the client to get them to realise that they have some underlying behavioural pattern that is preventing them from recovering. In psychological terms these health negating behavioural patterns are the basis of the phenomena known as 'secondary gain'. When working with a client to discover the nature of their patterns of secondary gain remember that it can sound as if you are saying that they *want* to be ill, which at a conscious level is hardly ever true. If you do not contextualise what you are saying you will create a great deal of very conscious, fiery resistance and probably lose the client as well. A situation that serves no one. You must give them an understanding of the nature of the sub-conscious mind, that what it does is always out of our conscious awareness.

Interestingly a 'habit pattern' can occur as the result of a long-standing conflict between a healing pattern and one that is negating it. Sometimes the behavioural pattern that was negating the healing pattern can have long since become inactive, but if this took a long time, say in excess of a few months, a third pattern can be set up. This would be a simple habit pattern which in effect is saying 'illness is my normal state of being'. If you have given a client a series of sessions and they do not seem to be improving, it does not necessarily mean that you have been doing the wrong thing or that your energy release work has been ineffective. It is more likely that you are being thwarted by a very deeply entrenched behavioural pattern. It is at this point that you must begin to work very directly with the sub-conscious mind patterns through deep analysis, affirmation work, or give them a good 'dutch uncle talk', to use Dr. Stone's phrase. Your approach is probably going to have to be very dynamic and fiery, but you must have the client's trust for this to work.

The reason that affirmations and the 'fiery dutch uncle' approach works is because one of the other basic qualities of the sub-conscious mind is its childlike impressionability. As a polarity therapist you have the edge over many other therapeutic approaches because you deal with life energy, which is the essence of real magic. After all you can create the most amazing sensations of movement, heat, and vibration in the body sometimes without even touching it. Even though the sub-conscious mind works with energy its own understanding of the laws which govern its action are often quite limited, particularly in the understanding that it can be influenced so readily and directly by someone else. However, the sub-conscious mind learns very quickly! In a sense, it seems to me that these behavioural patterns are intelligent, as individual segments of consciousness (or unconsciousness) that in some way have the capability to self regulate and adapt through a feedback mechanism. This is why the first two or perhaps three polarity sessions can be so effective, and why it can get more difficult as the sessions continue. Not as some people think because you are having to work more deeply, but because you are dealing with a very much more knowledgeable sub-conscious. You could say that the first couple of sessions slip in beneath the defenses because the sub-conscious patterns of secondary gain do not understand the nature of the enemy. To be able to maintain the therapeutic progress you as therapist-magician must have new spells to introduce as the therapy continues, and the artistry to come up with new and different ways to work with the life energy. As a polarity therapist it is reassuring to know that you can approach the work in so many different ways through touch, diet, exercise and counselling. As Dr. Stone himself did, there is even the possibility of using precious metals and crystals. Magic indeed!

In polarity therapy two of the basic principles are the hermetic laws 'as above, so below' and 'as within, so without'. In reading over the last few pages on the sub-conscious mind you will have noticed the allusion I made to the similarity between the sub-conscious mind and a computer system, and in fact I do believe there is a strong relationship between the two. I suspect the ability to create the computers we use today comes from the fact that our sub-conscious mind is the computer within, which we have now manifested as the electronic silicon-chip machines without. Indeed, how could we create something outside of ourselves that was not somehow already within us in some form or another?

As polarity therapists we are working to unblock the flow of life energy so that the healing patterns can work effectively. We do not need to decide in what way the energy should flow. It is the fundamental healing patterns stored in the memory of the sub-conscious mind that will determine that. However, we do need to have an awareness of all the things that might prevent those patterns from being effective. An understanding of the nature and functioning of the sub-conscious mind is invaluable for both yourself and your clients. Polarity therapy is as much a learning process for the client as it is a healing one. All polarity practitioners are health educators as well as therapists.

The nature of the conscious mind is quite different from that of the sub-conscious mind. The conscious mind is composed of all the psychological processes that you can be or are aware of: for example, your sense perceptions of both your body and the world around you and your ability to reason. It does not function independently of the sub-conscious mind. It relies on the sub-conscious to provide it with access to memory. Memories not just of earlier life experiences but memories concerning the manner in which the conscious sense perceptions and information about life absorbed at a conscious level can be processed. If we look at the computer analogy again then the sub-conscious mind is the data and programmes, and the conscious mind is the central processing unit; that part of the computer that processes, manipulates and modifies input or new data on the basis of existing patterns. It absorbs the new information and holds it in the short-term memory (ram). It also accesses the stored programme from the long-term memory and places it in the short-term memory. Then having both the new information and a pattern as to how it can be processed in the short-term memory, it manipulates or modifies the new information on the basis of this pattern.

As human beings we take in information and then manipulate it in various ways based on previous experience, and we call this 'thinking'. The way in which we think is based on previous experience and learning. Most of our thinking is done on the basis of patterns that are frequently referred to as 'beliefs'. Our biggest problem is that we do not review and modify our patterns of information processing — our 'beliefs' — often enough. We end up spending an inordinate amount of time on what is best described as distorted thinking; that is thinking that is inappropriate to our current life situation. This happens because most of us do not actually learn from our experience, as learning is not experiencing life and thinking about those experiences with a pattern of logic that was appropriate ten years ago. It is absorbing life experience and allowing this to modify our actual patterns of thinking. In computer terminology this is analogous to the point at which there is a recognition that the kind of information that you are having to deal with now requires a new programme that has greater built-in flexibility and power. A programme that is able to deal more adequately with the new input. In a computer system, if you input too much new information or information of a different nature from that which the programme is able to process, it will crash. It will just stop functioning. In a sense it is rather unfortunate that as human beings we are not as limited as a computer system. We have an *enormous* capacity for absorbing new experience and processing it by inappropriate beliefs before we crash. It can take us an amazing length of time before realising that there is a problem.

Distorted thinking on the basis of outmoded beliefs is a major therapeutic problem. How

44

many times have you heard a client make such statements as 'I am always ill', 'my relationships never work', 'nobody likes me', 'I never have any money', 'you won't be able to help me', 'my husband (wife) does not understand me', 'I am worthless', 'I never succeed at anything', 'I can't change my job', 'doing that will not help.' All these and many more that you hear every day are all examples of rigidity and distortion in the conscious mind. Always suspect distorted thinking when a client uses words like; can't, never, always, nobody. Words that imply limitation and negativity. You can always ascertain the amount of sub-conscious holding-on when working with a client to alter their way of thinking, by the degree of passion and emotionality with which they defend their old beliefs. As we all know, some beliefs are easily changed in the light of clearer logic or new experience, but I am sure you have all had experience of trying to change some aspect of yourself and your thinking in your own personal therapy and met a solid wall of emotional resistance which tells you that it is a pattern which your sub-conscious believes still has survival value.

Affirmations are a basic tool that can be used to change distorted patterns of thinking. I tend to think of them as new programmes for the mind-computer, as the affirmational process is in essence a re-programming technique. If we look at the structure of affirmations the first thing you will notice is that they are always stated in positive terms. Secondly, they are always phrased so as to be the opposite of an old belief. Thirdly, the constant internal repetition and the seeding of your environment with slips of paper with the affirmation written on them, creates a constant input of the new information to the conscious mind. It becomes memory resident, a piece of information that is always present in the short-term memory. Ultimately, because of this, it will be a modifying factor when the old belief is activated. In the long term it will be stored in the sub-conscious along with the old belief as a new parameter that will mean the old belief is now always modified when accessed, or that it will modify the old belief so much that it no longer exists in its original form.

Affirmations work best when you can inspire in the client a strong positive attitude towards the technique. This enlists the help of the sub-conscious mind. The best approach to getting a client to feel positive whilst doing the affirmations is to talk passionately about the possibilities that could open up in their life as a result of the changes in their attitudes and thinking. When teaching affirmations there is a real need for you to be positive all the time, even if the results are not manifesting for the client. Even if the final outcome is not the kind of change in the client's outer world as implicit in the technique, it is always possible to emphasise to them the positive internal attitudinal change that always occurs if you do an affirmation for any length of time. At the very least the expectant, hopeful attitude engendered is an excellent result.

In relation to illness and disease the conscious mind has an interesting role. In particular the aspect we call 'awareness' or conscious recognition. A person goes into therapy because they have a conscious awareness that they have a problem. They are aware either of pain and limited mobility or some form of emotional distress. There are of course certain kinds of diseases that do not impinge on conscious awareness until they are at quite an advanced stage, but this situation does not concern us here. As soon as one has an awareness of a problem it creates a response in your thinking. You evaluate your awareness of the problem against your previous experiences of a similar nature to see what you know about it, and to decide if it warrants further attention other than waiting for the body to heal itself or the emotions to calm down. If the problem persists for more than a short period of time your awareness of it will form the experience into a pattern to be stored in your long-term memory. Once this has happened the problem has already become a part of your ongoing reality. This is one reason why during a treatment, if I happen to press on a part of the client's body that is extremely tender, of which they were previously unaware, I pass off the almost inevitable questions of 'what is that?', 'what does that mean?', or 'what does that relate to?', with something like the following response: 'it is nothing, just a sore muscle', 'it is not important and it does not relate to anything', 'it's just a bit of local tension.' I do not want them to start worrying about other problems that were out of their awareness. Such worrying only makes them more difficult to resolve. If it is a problem that is out of their awareness just treat it along with the problem that they are aware of.

It is obvious from our look at mind and energy so far that memory plays a vital role. This role is nicely illustrated by a study done some years ago on people with chronic back trouble, people who said that they experienced almost constant pain. Firstly they found that in actual fact they were not in pain all the time but that sometimes were quite unaware of it. Secondly, if you asked them about the pain at a time when they were not actually feeling it, they would place their hand on their back and re-evoke the experience of the pain from memory. I see memory as a separate entity from mind. It is a separate storehouse for both inner and outer life experiences. Memory can be accessed by all the different levels of mind. Our whole identity is based upon memory. We are the sum of all our previous thoughts and experiences. A great deal of the fragmentation of character and identity that we experience is caused because we can only access a limited proportion of our total life experience at any one time. Many disease states and general imbalance are prolonged due to the client consciously accessing their memory concerning the particular problem. Part of the process of recovery is to no longer re-evoke your memory of the problem. It is quite a common experience for a client to say, in response to your question concerning how they feel about the problem that you have been treating them for, that they were not aware of it so it must be getting better. In part this is due to the fact that quite probably they are in fact getting better, but that also they are no longer interested or even able to access their memory of the discomfort that they felt.

The concept of awareness and memory that I have outlined above is perhaps most simply elucidated in the following situation. A teenager who has had facial spots for some months will wash their face at night and perhaps apply some form of skin treatment before retiring, in the hope that the treatment will remove the spots. When they wake up in the morning it is quite possible that their skin may have cleared significantly, but because this has not happened in the previous weeks they have built up a belief that has become stored in their memory that the spots will probably still be there in the morning. As they lie in bed before either touching their face or looking in the mirror they are often caught up in a number of conflicting thoughts; a hopeful belief that the spots may be gone because the doctor or therapist had said that they would probably take some weeks to go, and a conflicting fearful one based upon weeks of experiencing little or no change every time they look in the mirror. In this situation memory is both supporting and negating the healing process. The question is, which of the thoughts is being enacted by the sub-conscious mind, as that will determine the actual situation. There is always the involvement of the sub-conscious and conscious minds as well as memory in all disease and imbalance.

The pattern of energy that relates directly to the conscious mind is the spirals of energy that radiate from the umbilicus. Dr. Stone called this particular energy pattern 'evolutionary energy' because it is the conscious mind that is the aspect of mind that is constantly seeking new experience and growth. The pattern of energy is a constantly expanding spiral which is but a reflection of the nature of the conscious mind, which is itself always seeking expansion, a broadening of its horizons. As all disease and imbalance involves some form of conscious awareness and distorted thinking, there is always going to be some degree of disturbance in the umbilical spirals of energy. As I pointed out, the sub-conscious and conscious minds work together, it is important to establish a functioning balance between the energy patterns that relate to the sub-conscious mind and those of the conscious mind. This can be done by tying in the umbilical spirals of energy to the chakra system. My perception is that the energy that emanates from the umbilicus is of a different octave from that of the caduceus and chakra system, and that the umbilicus is not the same as the fire chakra (see Appendix I, page 130).

The super-conscious mind is that aspect of mind that is fundamentally linked to, or is synonymous with, the soul. It is the organising or seed pattern. In our analogy of the mind as a computer the super-conscious mind is the actual operator, the person who chose the system in the first place and who ultimately determines the input. In my experience the only disease states that are related to the super-conscious mind are major or life threatening illnesses such as cancer. If a person indulges in excessive amounts of distorted thinking and does not adequately utilise the learning capabilities that they have, and refuses to seek out the true meaning of life, from the operator's point of view the information they put in is being badly processed. At a certain point the operator is going to get so frustrated by the computer's inability to deal appropriately with the input that the only choice he has is to shut down the system. He would then either restart the system in the hopes that it was just a temporary bug, or would have to consider creating a completely new programme with which to process the input, but this would mean deleting the old programme.

In human terms, sometimes the only way to shift somebody from such an inappropriate approach to life is that they would have to experience an illness of truly life-changing proportions; a terminal illness. I have noticed in my work with clients suffering from this kind of problem that the ones who survive are the ones who were prepared to change their whole life; to change their diet, their job, their relationships, their way of thinking and so forth, right down almost to the smallest details. As I mentioned earlier, the power of the mind is such that it is able to hold many conflicting thoughts and beliefs as well as being able to struggle with many of life's difficulties before finally crashing. Sadly, from a soul point of view, the length of time taken for a person to come to this realisation is often too long, and through its ability to interact with the pattern body or etheric body it will create a situation whereby some life-threatening disease is going to manifest, thereby giving the person a very powerful signal to re-evaluate their life.

It is the superconscious mind through the etheric body that defines the pattern of flow of all the other frequencies of life energy in the body. The superconscious mind energy is a higher octave of energy again than either the chakra system or the umbilical spiral. It probably functions in a somewhat similar way to the magnetic bottles that were developed by modern atomic physicists to contain plasma, a highly energised form of matter that exists in the heart of the sun. It is the etheric or pattern body; in effect one very high intensity energy field defining the shape of another highly energised field. There has been some confusion concerning the meaning of the word 'etheric body' since it was first used by the theosophists at the end of the last century. It is not related to the throat or ether chakra. It is the phrase they used to express the idea that for anything to flow in a certain pattern it must first have something through which to flow, and secondly the actual shape of the conducting medium would define the pattern of that flow. For example, if you want water to flow in a zig-zag pattern you simply dig a zig-zag shaped ditch and then channel some water in to it.

47

The boundary of the etheric body is the same as the boundary of the health or physical aura which very definitely follows the contour of the physical body, which is why they called it the etheric *body* and sometimes the etheric double. They also used the term 'etheric energy' as their generic name for all the different frequencies of life energy that flow within the etheric body. The overall shape of all the different frequencies of life energy was called the aura. Over the last twenty years, as the concept of life energy and energy balancing has spread, many older texts have been re-issued and people who have read them have ascribed their own interpretation to the archaic and scientifically outdated concepts contained within them. These same people have subsequently written books on healing and used these terms with different meanings, adding to the general confusion. I have no doubt that Dr. Stone studied all of the early theosophical texts by Leadbeater et al. My study of the places in his writings where he uses these phrases leads me to believe he did not always use them in their original meaning. This can be very confusing, particularly if you are familiar with the original usage and meaning of the terms.

I have over the last few years discovered the pattern of energy flow in the human body that I feel is intimately linked to the superconscious mind. A pattern of energy not mapped in Dr. Stone's pioneering work. It is the energy pattern that sustains the etheric double. I have also discovered a number of ways of working with this pattern, but it is not within the scope of this book to explore this area in any further detail.

7   Energy Balancing Techniques

Ear Treatments

The ears relate to the ether element as well as being located in the fire element oval. The ear canal is the positive pole of the centre of gravity in the body which is at the umbilicus. The ear canal has the same relationship to the head as the umbilicus has to the body, and this suggests the possibility of treating any disturbance in the head by polarising it to the ears. It is also possible to polarise the ear to any other part of the body. The diagnostic areas as represented in the ear are: the upper ear relating to the area above the diaphragm, the middle ear relating to the abdominal area, and the ear lobe relating to the pelvis. Any of these areas that show redness or discoloration are diagnostic indicators of a disturbance in the organs represented by that location. Dr. Stone recommended some specific directions for the application of a gentle force when working the ears. However, I have found that thinking of the centre of the ear as the hub of a bicycle wheel and the spokes of the wheel as representing all the different lines of force to check, it is in fact relevant to check them all. Working the ear canal is the key to releasing the cranial bones because of the influence it has on the sphenoid bone.

TECHNIQUE 1
Client is on his back
Step 1. Stand at the client's head.
    2. Place the earth fingers in the ear canals, keeping the fingers relaxed and open (Fig. 6).

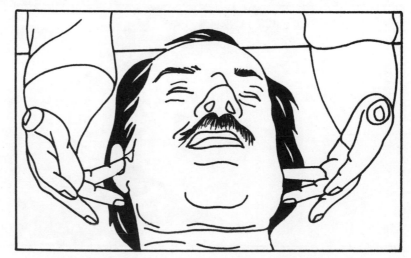

Fig. 6

3. Test for tenderness in the ear canal by gently pulling (or pushing) in the directions of force as described in the above text (Fig. 7).
4. Once you have found a sore line of force, stimulate the ears alternately by applying a gentle pressure in the same direction through the earth fingers (a wiggling movement), until the tenderness has gone.
5. Release all other lines of force that are sore.

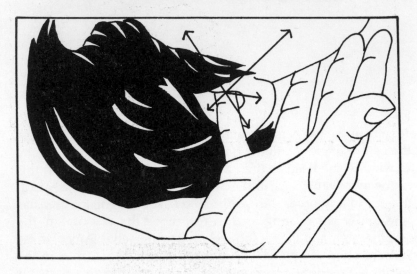

Fig. 7

TECHNIQUE 2
Client is on his back
Step 1. Stand at the client's head.
    2. Place your air fingers into the ear canal (Fig. 8).
    3. Grip the tragus (the small lobe) of each ear between your air fingers and thumbs (Fig. 9).
    4. Stimulate each tragus by firmly stretching and rotating it in different directions for about 1 minute. Hold and feel for the energy.

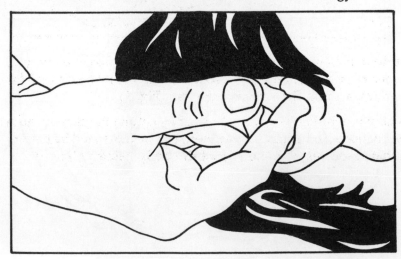

Fig. 8

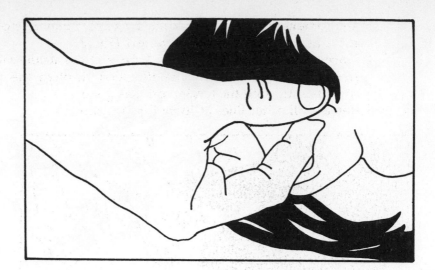

Fig. 9

TECHNIQUE 3

Client is on his back

Step 1. Stand at the client's head.

2. Place your thumbs in the ears (Fig. 10).

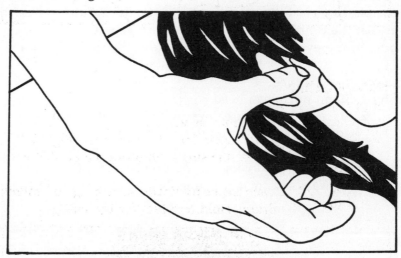

Fig. 10

3. Using the fingers to grip the outside of the ears and using the thumbs as a fulcrum, stretch and pull the ear over the thumbs for about 1 minute. Hold and feel for energy. Continue working around the whole of the ear (Fig. 11).

Note: The effectiveness of the above techniques can be enhanced by getting the client to hum at a pitch that gives a response in the ears. In fact any treatment can be enhanced by getting the client to hum at a pitch that resonates with the part of the body being polarised.

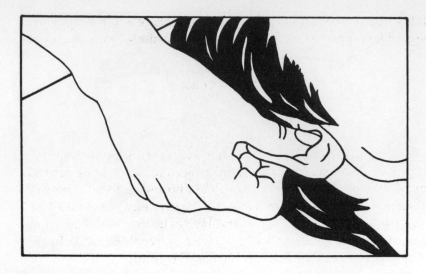

Fig. 11

Eye/Digestion Treatment

This is an excellent release for both the function of the eyes and the digestion as a whole. The occipital area is the motor release area for the eyes as well as being a reflex to the abdominal area at the umbilical level. The orbital ridge is a reflex to the diaphragm and is the positive pole of the eyes which are part of the fire astrological triad (eyes, solar plexus, thighs).

Client is on his back
Step 1. Stand at client's head.
   2. Place your right fire finger at the left orbital corner near the bridge of the nose and your left air finger on the occipital ridge ¼ inch to the left of the spine.
   3. Stimulate alternately for 1 minute. Hold and feel for energy.
   4. Continue polarising all the points along the occipital and orbital ridge working outwards ½ inch at a time. Fig. 12 shows the technique at mid-point on the two ridges.

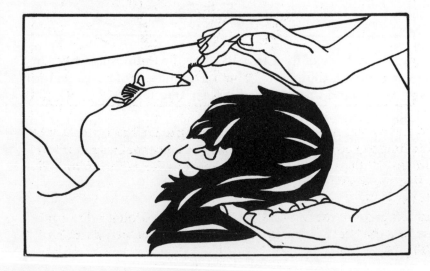

Fig. 12

5. Repeat on the right side using the left air finger on the orbital ridge and the right fire finger on the occipital ridge. This whole treatment can be done with diagonal contacts.

Cranial Moulding

Cranial moulding is an approach to cranial release that does not rely on working any specific rhythms of cranial energetic pulsations. Instead it just simply seeks to release the cranial sutures and energy in a general way so that the cerebro-spinal impulse is freed. The self regulating nature of the cerebro-spinal system ensures that the energy released comes into balance of its own accord. It releases the fire element oval and the circulation of the prana in the cerebro-spinal fluid. The cranial sutures need only a light touch to free them when fixed, just as a pendulum needs only a light touch to set it in motion. Be gentle.

Client is seated
(The height of the stool on which the client sits should allow their head to be at your chest level)
Step 1. Stand behind the client.
2. Place both hands over the client's ears, fingers pointing towards the top of the head, so that the heel of the palm hooks the mastoid process and the angle of the jaw on each side (Fig. 13).

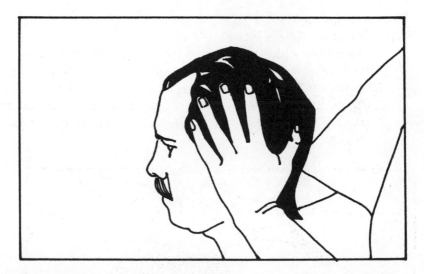

Fig. 13

3. Apply a *slight* upward and inward lift on the head as if trying to lift it away from the shoulders, at the same time as you are gently squeezing it. Once the head is at full lift apply a gentle vibration through the hands for ten seconds. Relax the lift for ten seconds and repeat this sequence 3 or 4 times.
4. Stand on the client's left side.
5. Place the heel of your left palm so that it is hooked beneath the orbital ridge over the bridge of the nose, and the heel of your right palm hooks the central portion of the occipital ridge (Fig. 14).

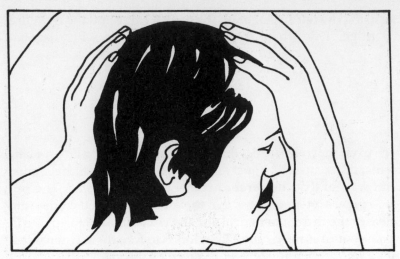

Fig. 14

6. Lift, squeeze and vibrate as in step 3. Repeat 3 or 4 times, resting between each lift.
7. Stay on the client's left side.
8. Place your left hand so that the heel of the palm hooks beneath the left outer edge of the orbital ridge, and the heel of your right palm hooks beneath the right mastoid process (Fig. 15).

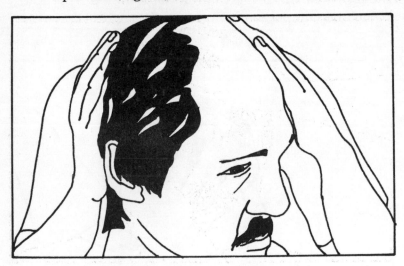

Fig. 15

9. Lift, squeeze and vibrate exactly as in step 6.
10. Stand on the client's right side.
11. Repeat steps 8 and 9. This time the contacts are on the right outer orbital ridge and left mastoid process.
12. Stand behind the client.
13. Place the heels of the palms over the temples with the fingers overlapping on the forehead (Fig. 16).
14. Apply a gentle squeezing movement to the client's temples, alternately increasing and decreasing the pressure every few seconds for about 1 minute.
15. Ask the client to lie down on the table and stand on their right side.

54

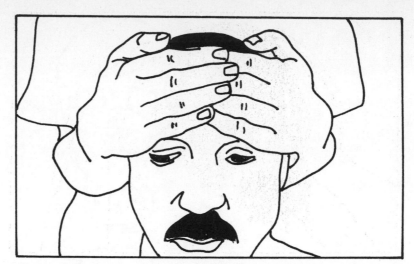

Fig. 16

16. Place your right thumb over their left cheek bone and allow the palm to mould to the face, and the heel of your left palm over their forehead just above the right eye (Fig. 17).
17. Apply a *slight* downward and outward stretch and then vibrate the cheek contact for about 30 seconds.
18. Repeat on the opposite side from right cheek to left forehead.

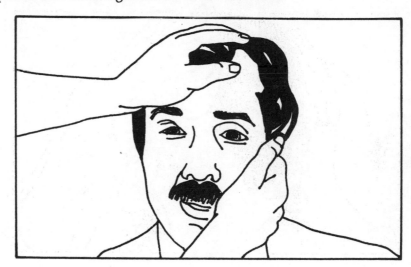

Fig. 17

Cranial Relationships

Fig. 18 shows how the skull, symbolising the creative mind patterns, steps down through the various oval fields of the body. It is a representation of consciousness pervading the body and setting up harmonic relationships in the process. It shows how the energy of the central nervous system enervates the body. The poles of the central nervous system are the cranium as the positive pole, the shoulder area as the neutral pole and the pelvis as the negative pole. The figure shows various relationships between the head and neck, head and chest, head and abdomen and head and pelvis. It also gives a basic proportional relationship between all

55

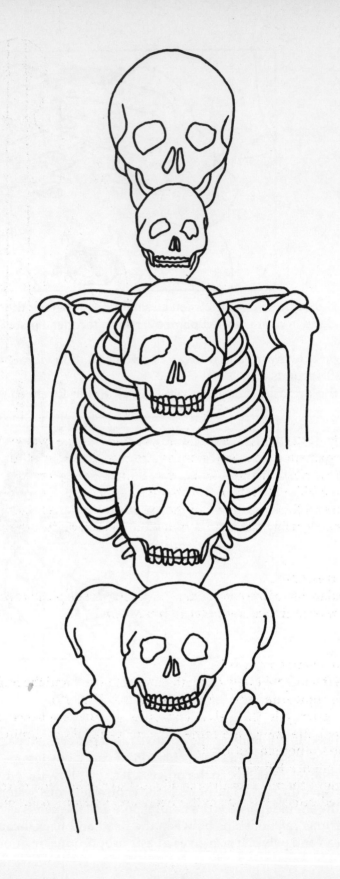

Fig. 18

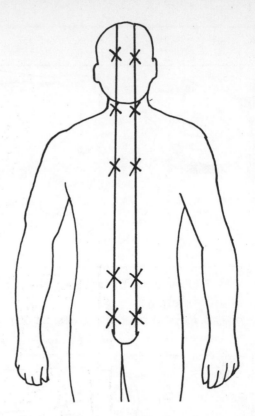

Fig. 19

of the five oval fields in the body. For example the pupil of the eye, which lies on the air current line, in approximately the centre of the fire oval, has four other nodal points that have powerful reflex relationships to it, the points being on the air current line approximately in the middle of each of the other four oval fields. These points are shown in Fig. 19. Therefore, an excellent treatment for the eyes is to place the fingertips over the eye to be treated and polarise it, using alternate stimulation, to each of the other four nodal points in turn.

CRANIAL/PELVIC BALANCE
This treatment is a balancing of the central nervous system at its positive and negative poles, and is an excellent way to finish any polarity treatment.

Client is on his back
Step 1. Stand on the client's right side.
2. Place your left hand obliquely along the line of the jaw, and the fingers of your right hand on the right side of the symphysis pubis (Fig. 20).
3. Feel for the energy in the pelvis and once you have a sense of its rhythm or vibration, rock the jaw to the same rhythm taking about 2 minutes altogether.
4. Repeat on the other side of the body.
5. Stay on the client's left side.
6. Place your right thumb over the maxilla just to the left side of the nose, with the fingers spread out on the side of the head, and your left hand cups the right iliac crest.

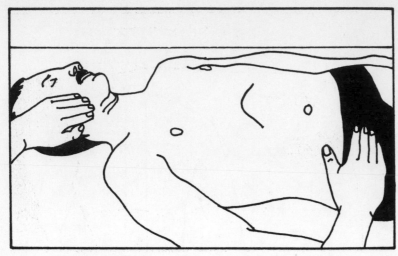

Fig. 20

7. Stimulate by rocking the iliac crest for 1-2 minutes. Hold and feel for the energy.

8. Repeat on the other side of the body (Fig. 21).

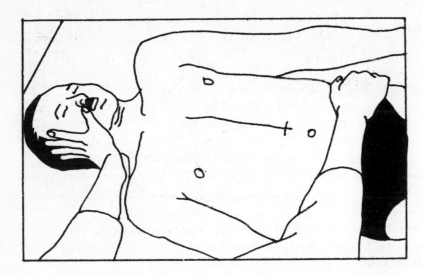

Fig. 21

9. Stay on the client's right side.

10. Place the left hand over the forehead and the right hand between the iliac crests (Fig. 22).

11. Rock the pelvic contact *very* softly, the range of movement is no more than ¼ inch, for 1-2 minutes. Hold and feel for energy.

12. Move the left hand slowly from the forehead and gently grip the bridge of the nose between the thumb and air finger. Peel the right hand slowly off the pelvis until you just have the outer edge of the palm left in contact (Fig. 23).

13. Stimulate the pelvis through the edge of the right palm as in step 11. Take the hands slowly off the body when finished.

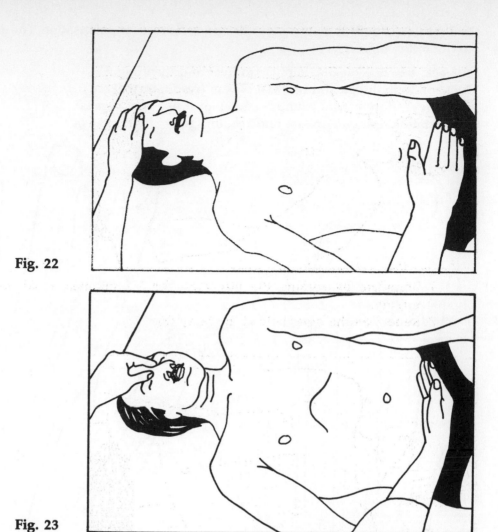

Fig. 22

Fig. 23

Note: The cranial/pelvic bone relationships upon which this treatment is based are:
Jaw — Symphysis pubis
Parietal bones — Innominate bones
Maxilla — Inguinal ligament
Frontal bone — Lower abdomen
Nasal bone — Mid-point in pelvic oval

Heart Therapy

The nature of a specific heart problem can be ascertained by checking for tenderness between the tendon interspaces of the left hand and foot, as well as checking for any distortions of the air, fire and water fingers. Fig. 24 shows the location of the tendon interspaces marked as areas 1, 2, 3 and 4. These particular areas are horizontal reflex areas and are useful both as diagnostic indicators and areas for polarisation. The areas correspond to the following organs.

1. Neck, brachial plexus, impulse to liver and diaphragm.
2. Diaphragm, lungs and brachial plexus (respiratory organs).
3. Kidneys, duodenum, jejunum and colon (digestive organs).
4. Prostate, uterus, perineum and rectum (generative organs).

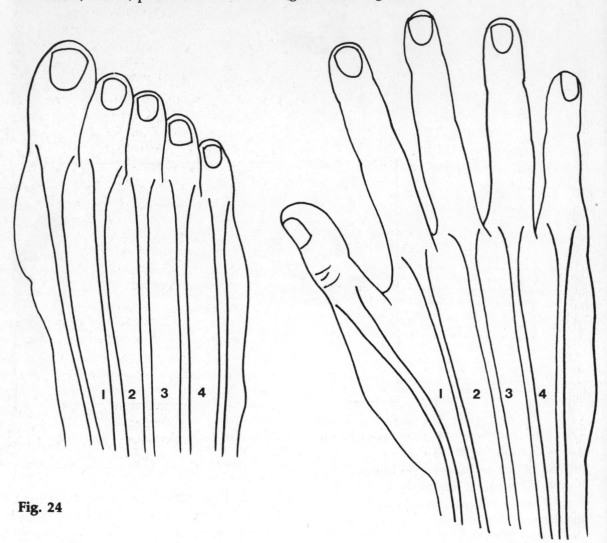

Fig. 24

Note: These areas and correspondences are the same on both left and right hands and feet.

The particular joint to check in the air, fire and water fingers is the first joint in each. The air finger is the true polarity reflex to the heart. When it is sore, in cases of heart trouble, then the air element is being over stressed and rest from mental, emotional strain is most important. It is indicative of a hypertension as the main factor. Soreness of tendon interspace 1 is also indicative of this kind of problem being the neck area, which is the link between the head

60

and the heart. When the first joint of the fire finger or tendon interspace 2 is sore, then it is the warmth in the circulation that is in trouble due to poor digestion and the probable accumulation of fatty deposits in the arteries and veins. When the first joint of the water finger and tendon interspace 3 is sore, then it is the watery matrix of the heart structure and the impulse for it to pump that are in trouble. The same relationships are true of the air, fire and water toes and tendon interspaces of the right foot. Remember the feet show chronic energy blocks and the hands acute energy blocks.

Client is on his back
Step 1. Stand at the client's feet.
   2. Polarise the first joints of the air, fire and water toes on both feet. Begin polarising both air toes simultaneously by gently pulling and squeezing them for 1 minute or until any tenderness has gone. Then continue with the fire and water toes in the same way.
   3. Polarise the tendon interspaces 1, 2 and 3 on both feet. Grip each foot between your thumb and fingers so that the thumb is underneath the foot and the fingers lie in the tendon interspace. Begin with tendon interspace 1 (Fig. 25). Stimulate by rhythmically squeezing the sore areas for 1 minute or until the tenderness

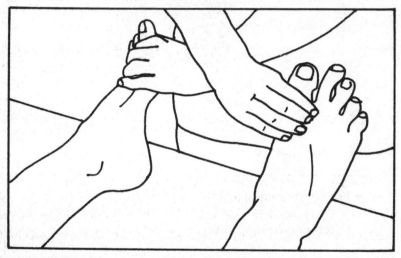

Fig. 25

disappears. It is sometimes easier to do this technique with the arms crossed.
   4. Polarise the fingers and tendon interspaces in the hands in the same way. See Fig. 26 for the tendon interspace grip on the hands.
   5. Release the brachial plexus on both sides.
   6. Stand on the client's right side.
   7. Place your right thumb at the tip of the sternum just beneath the xiphoid process, and the left hand grips the right shoulder with the thumb beneath the clavicle (Fig. 27).
   8. Rhythmically squeeze the muscles over the right shoulder and alternate this with a directional contact of the thumb up under the ribs towards the right shoulder. Work along the line of the right lower ribs, releasing any tender areas. In some cases, due to the amount of tension, the little finger has to be used instead of the thumb.

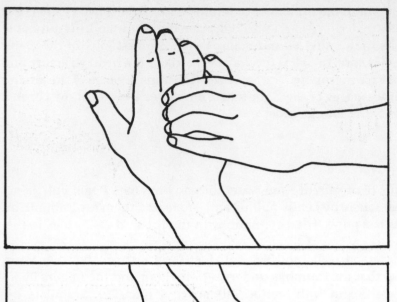

Fig. 26

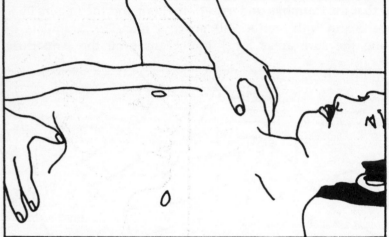

Fig. 27

9. Staying on the same side of the client's body, reach across to the left shoulder with your left hand and free any tender area along the left lower ribs, using the same techniques as in step 8.

Note: Steps 5-9 are specifically aimed at releasing any tension or spasticity in the diaphragm. The diaphragm is the most important muscle in relation to heart function, and its balanced functioning is a vital factor to achieve in any heart therapy. Details on the specifics of releasing the brachial plexus are in the book *Polarity Therapy, the power that heals* by Alan Siegel (Prism Press).

10. Still on the right side of the client's body, place your right thumb once more at the xiphoid process, pointing upwards. To stimulate the heart function the left thumb is placed over the third eye, with the fingers on the section of the line of cardiac stability that is above the left ear (Fig. 28). The cardiac stability is shown in Fig. 28a.
11. Stimulate the cardiac stability with a gentle movement of the left fingers, as you hold the right thumb contact steady for about 1 minute.
12. To relax the heart function the left hand is laid along the line of the left side of the

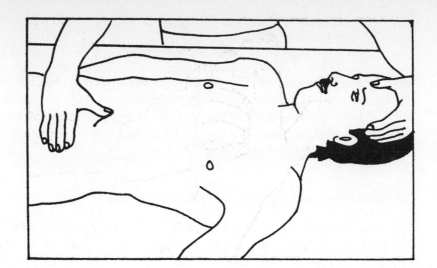

Fig. 28

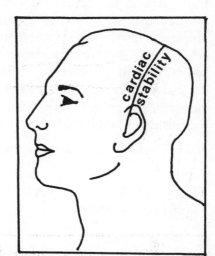

Fig. 28a

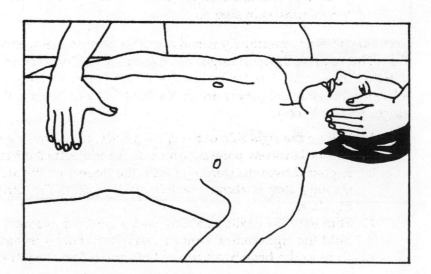

Fig. 29

jaw, and the thumb of the right hand at the xiphoid process is directed towards the jaw contact (Fig. 29).

13. There is no stimulation in this technique. It is a satvic hold.

Note: The cardiac stability (Fig. 28a) is a cranial control reflex for heart function. It runs along the line of the left side of the jaw, through the ear, and then parallels the line of the frontal/ parietal bone sutures at about the middle of the parietal bone. The upper section of the line is the contact area for tonifying heart action, the lower section for sedating it. Tonify or sedate the heart according to the client's needs.

Contacts With and Against Surface Current Flow

These techniques are used for releasing local energy blocks anywhere on the body. One or two hands may be used when applying the technique, whichever gives the best response. The main energetic effect of these techniques is created by the directional impulse behind them, not on the actual polarity of your contacts. All these techniques are done using the whole body to give momentum to the technique. The nature of the contacts is a low amplitude pulse. It is important to maintain an overall relaxation throughout the whole body when applying these techniques. Contacts that are applied with the current flow are soothing in their effect, and contacts against the current flow are stimulating. Contacts with the current flow are used where there is heat, pain and inflammation, and contacts against current flow are used when there is muscular spasm, paralysis or excess tension. In all the techniques you should vary the angle of application until you get the best response.

Note: The following three techniques are done *with the current flow*.

TECHNIQUE 1
Client is on his front

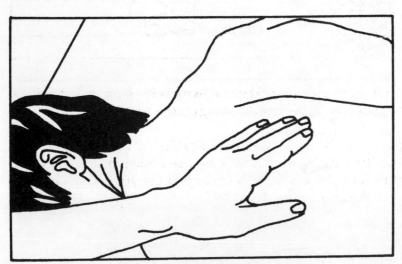

Fig. 30

Step 1. Stand on the client's left side.
2. Place your left palm on the upper back at a 45 degree angle (Fig. 30).

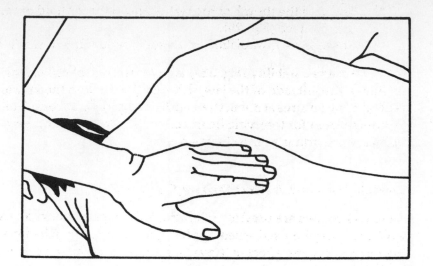

Fig. 31

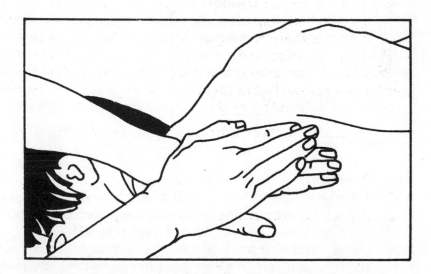

Fig. 32

3. Twist your left hand until the fingers are pointing downwards, whilst maintaining a firm but relaxed contact with the skin, thereby taking up the slack in the underlying tissues (Fig. 31).
4. Firm your contact by placing the right hand on top of the left hand (Fig. 32).
5. Shifting your weight to the balls of your feet, pulse the client's body by rocking backwards and forwards for 1-2 minutes. Make sure you use your whole body to achieve the pulsing, not just your arms (Fig. 33).

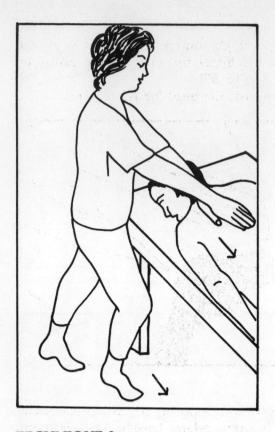

Fig. 33

TECHNIQUE 2

Client is on his back

Step 1. Stand on the client's right side.

    2. Place your left hand over the client's right lower abdomen so that the fingers over the pubic bone are pointing downwards, and your right hand is on the upper thigh with the fingers also pointing downwards (Fig. 34).

    3. Using your whole body as in step 5 of technique 1, pulse downwards towards the feet for 1-2 minutes. Make sure your hands do not slide over the skin.

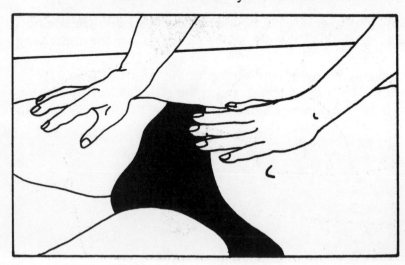

Fig. 34

4. Stand on the client's left side.
5. Place your left hand on the client's left upper thigh, fingers pointing upwards, and your right hand on the abdomen so that the finger tips are pushing gently up underneath the floating ribs on the left side (Fig. 35).
6. As in Step 3 pulse your hands upwards towards the head for 1-2 minutes.

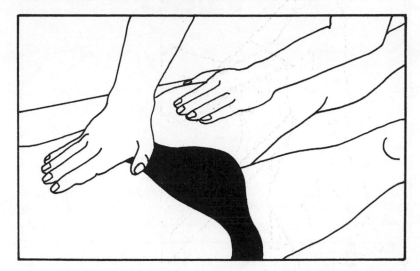

Fig. 35

TECHNIQUE 3
This particular technique polarises the spine by creating an opposing stretch in the muscles on either side. It can be done anywhere along the spine where tension, pain or spasm exists.

Client is on his front
Step 1. Stand on the client's left side.
2. Place your left hand over the spine at a 45 degree angle so that the palm is covering the lower dorsal vertebrae, and place your right palm over the top as a support (Fig. 36).

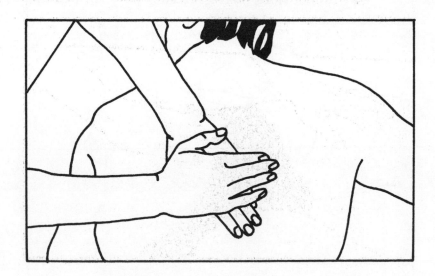

Fig. 36

3. Applying firm pressure twist your hands anticlockwise (Fig. 37).
4. Holding the muscles under tension, pulse your hands upwards towards the head by using a rocking movement of your whole body until the muscles relax. Vibratory impulses may be used instead.

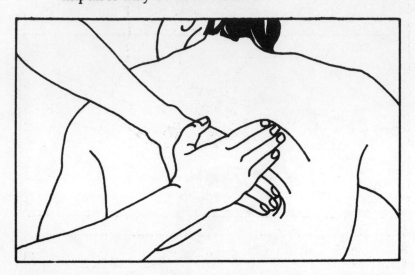

Fig. 37

Muscular Drainage by Opposing Forces (The 'S' Technique)

This technique was recommended by Dr. Stone as one of the simplest and most effective ways of draining a muscle of stagnant material. It is best done against the local current flow as a stimulating contact.

Client is on his front
Step 1. Stand on the client's left side.
2. Place your right thumb on the left side of a tense muscle fibre and your left thumb on the right side. The tensest muscles are often near the spine (Fig. 38).
3. Push your right thumb upwards and your left thumb downwards, making sure that they do not slide, thereby creating an 'S' shaped fold in the tissues (Fig. 39).

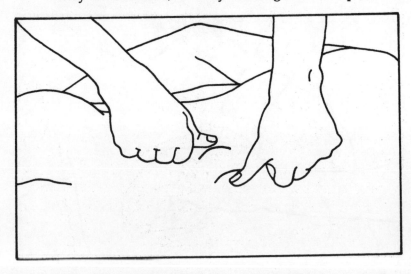

Fig. 38

4. The same basic technique can be done horizontally on the body (Fig. 40). It can also be done using the whole hand (Fig. 41).

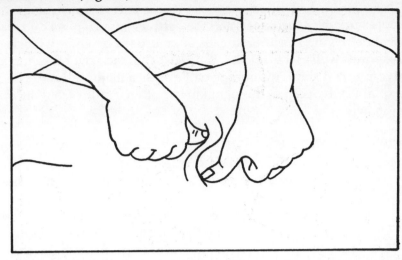

Fig. 39

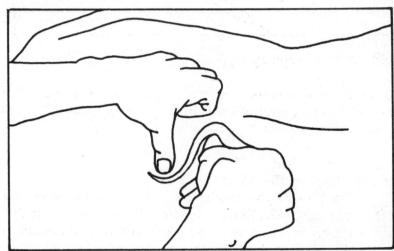

Fig. 40

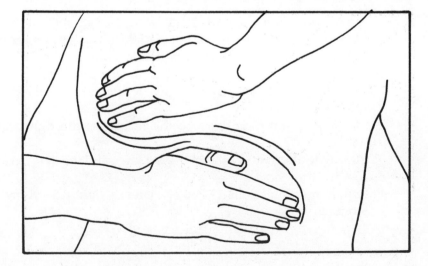

Fig. 41

Digestive Treatment

This is an earth element treatment. It uses part of the astrological triad of the earth element as represented by the knees, and the earth element's physical area of function, the abdominal oval field. Pain in either knee is often caused by energy blocks in the liver or stomach and responds well to this release. It also uses contacts over the Poupart's ligament, the base of the five-pointed star. This energy pattern has a major influence on the digestive system. It also explains why pain in the right knee is often a reflex from the opposite side of the body, the stomach.

Client is on his back
Step 1. Stand on the client's left side.
    2. Place your left hand over the left knee and the fingertips of your right hand over the Poupart's ligament on the left side (Fig. 42).
    3. Stimulate alternately by rocking the knee gently and working your fingers gently down in to the pelvis, then up towards the opposite shoulder with a scooping movement for 1-2 minutes. Hold and feel for the energy.

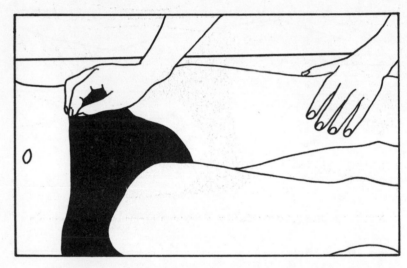

Fig. 42

    4. Move your left hand to the Poupart's ligament on the left side and your right hand to the liver area on the opposite side of the body. The fingertips of the right hand can be placed just up underneath the floating ribs on the right side if required (Fig. 43).
    5. Stimulate the Poupart's ligament as in step 3, and alternate it with a gentle rocking of the liver area up towards the right shoulder alternately for 1-2 minutes. Hold and feel for the energy.
    6. Move your left hand back to the left knee, the right stays on the liver area (Fig. 44).
    7. Stimulate alternately by rocking the knee and the liver area for 1-2 minutes. Hold and feel for the energy.
    8. Repeat manipulations 1-7 on the client's right side. Remember to cross over to the stomach.

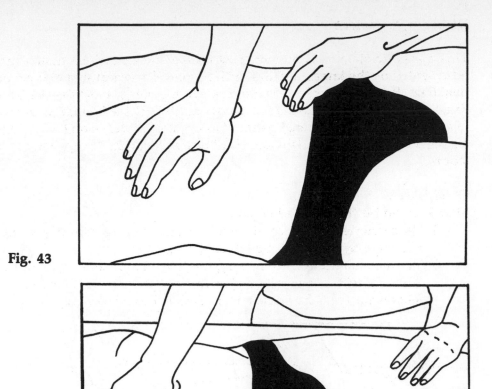

Fig. 43

Fig. 44

Balancing by Contour

Balancing by Contour is the name given by Dr. Stone to treating blocked areas in the body on the basis of the hermetic principle of correspondence. I also use the term 'symmetry of form' as an alternative title for this kind of balancing work. In essence, it is those areas of the body that have similar contour or shape with a definite reflex relationship to each other. The sore spots in a particular area can be released by polarising them to points in other areas of similar shape. Fig. 45 shows dotted areas as contact points in the pelvic girdle below relating to similar points in the shoulder girdle above. From the elemental point of view, releasing buttocks and shoulders is a balancing of the air and water elements, and releasing the strain in these areas results in a definite improvement in the quality of movement. This treatment is also a balancing of the parasympathetic nervous system, because the upper gluteal muscles are supplied by the sacral parasympathetic nerves and the neck and shoulder muscles by the vagus and the spinal accessory nerves, which are also a part of the parasympathetic nervous system.

71

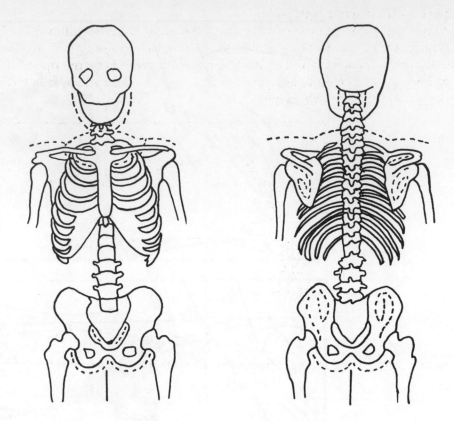

Fig. 45

Client is on his front
Step1. Stand on the client's left side.
    2. Using your right thumb find the sorest spot over the left buttock, and with your left thumb the sorest spot over the left scapula.
    3. Holding the sore spot over the scapula with your left thumb, stimulate the sore area on the buttock with your right. Try using different directions of gentle force on the buttock contact until the tenderness in both areas is gone. You may also use alternate stimulation if you wish (Fig. 46).

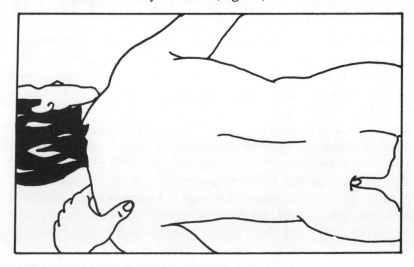

Fig. 46

4. Repeat on the client's right side.
5. In some cases the stress and strain may cross diagonally to the other side of the body, in which case the contacts are from buttock to opposite shoulder. The release of the buttock to the muscles between the spine and the scapula on the opposite side is an excellent way of freeing the diaphragm. Use the same procedure as in steps 2 - 4 but making diagonal contacts (Fig. 47).

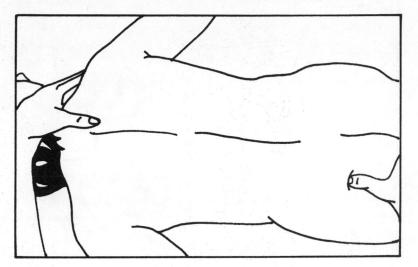

Fig. 47

Breast Treatment

This treatment, which is very useful in treating lumps and stagnation in the breasts, is a balancing of the posterior motor reflex areas of the water element. The scapula area is the motor pole of the breasts, the buttocks provide the push (motor action) to the genitals, and the calves provide the motive power to the feet. The actual areas for treatment are shown in Fig. 48.

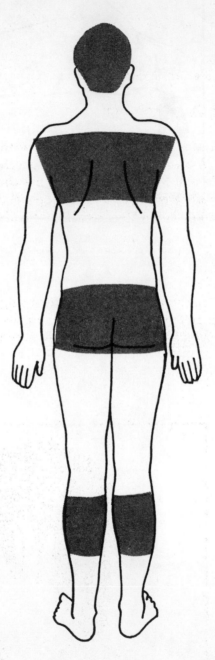

Fig. 48

Client is on their front

Step1. Stand on the client's left side.

2. Place the left hand palm down over the left buttock, and the right hand palm down over the calf area, fingers pointing towards the head. The contact areas are as shaded in Fig. 48.

3. Stimulate by simultaneously rocking both contacts in a headward direction for 1-2 minutes.

4. Move the left palm up to the left scapula and the right palm to the left buttock.

5. Stimulate as in step 3.

6. Leave the left palm on the scapula and move the right palm back down to the calf area.

7. Stimulate as in step 3.

8. Repeat on the right side of the client's body.

Seated Release of Neck and Dorsal Vertebrae

This is a countryside technique for releasing all the vertebrae from the top of the spine down to the ninth dorsal vertebrae. A countryside technique is a technique that is done when you do not have access to a table and have to work with the client seated. It is an excellent manipulation for freeing vertebral fixation. It uses diagonal contacts to activate the deep currents down the spine. The hold on the head stabilises the client's body as well as centrally positioning the atlas.

Client is seated

Step1. Stand behind the client.

2. Wrap your right arm around the front of the client's right shoulder and place your right hand on the side of their head, so that the ear lies between the water and fire fingers (Fig. 49) and the ball of your left thumb at the side of a fixed and tender vertebrae.

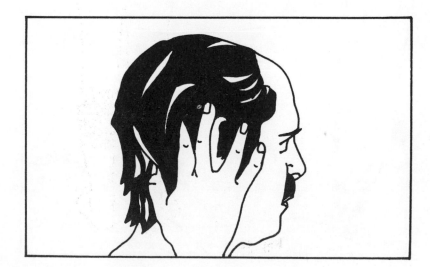

Fig. 49

3. Stimulate the vertebrae by vibrating your left thumb in towards the centreline of the body for about 1 minute, or until the tenderness has gone (Fig. 50).
4. Treat all other sore vertebrae in the same way. Treat both sides of the spine if necessary.

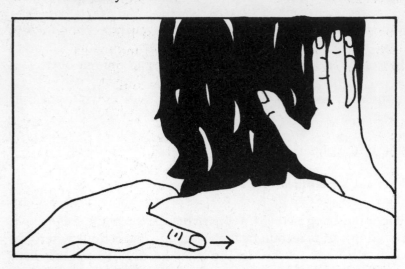

Fig. 50

Lower Pelvic Release

Tension and soreness in the lower rectus abdominus and pyramidalis muscles is usually indicative of disturbance in the underlying organs (the bladder, uterus, prostate, or rectum). Releasing the muscle tension above improves the functioning of the organs below. This technique can also be used as a powerful sacral re-positioning manipulation in cases of a sacral distortion that is not reacting favourably to vibratory techniques.

Client is on his back
Step1. Stand on the client's right side.
    2. Place your left hand underneath the back of the neck and occiput, and the ball of your right thumb flat over the tense muscle fibres just above the symphysis pubis (Fig. 51).

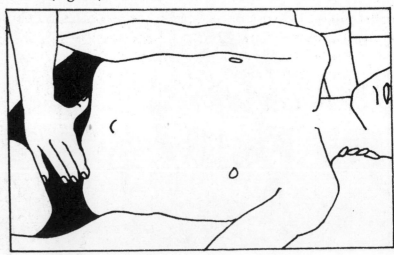

Fig. 51

3. Ask the client to breathe in, and as they breathe out lift upwards on the neck as you hold the thumb steady over the tense muscles. Hold the stretch for a moment and then let the upper body down gently. Allow a short period of relaxation and repeat the sequence three more times (Fig. 52).

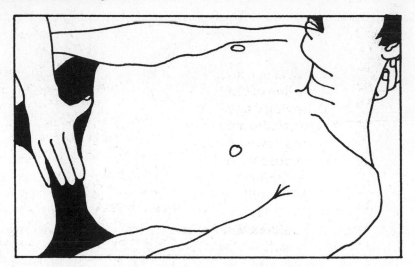

Fig. 52

Note: When using this as a sacral correction, the thumb contact is on the anterior sacral base side of the pelvis over the middle area of the Poupart's ligament.

Stimulating Sensory Current Flow

This is an ether treatment because it works on the joints of the body. It seeks to stimulate the return or sensory flow of energy in the body from the circumference back to the centre, and so has a balancing effect in relation to the motor currents of energy. However, it is my feeling that when Dr. Stone talks about the centre and circumference, in this case he is referring to the umbilicus and the spiral of energy that radiates from it. I see it as being a treatment that slows down or balances an excess of activity in the umbilical spirals of energy. In fact the first contact points on the hands and feet are reflex points to the umbilicus. It is very useful in a situation where a client is pushing out far too much energy in frenetic activity; for example, in the frantic days just before Christmas. It can be done on the front or the back of the body as required. From a symptomatic point of view, I have found this treatment to be of enormous benefit in cases of rheumatoid arthritis and for stopping the hot flushes associated with the female menopause. Fig. 53 shows the contact areas as points above and below the line of flexion of a joint in a diamond-shaped area of action.

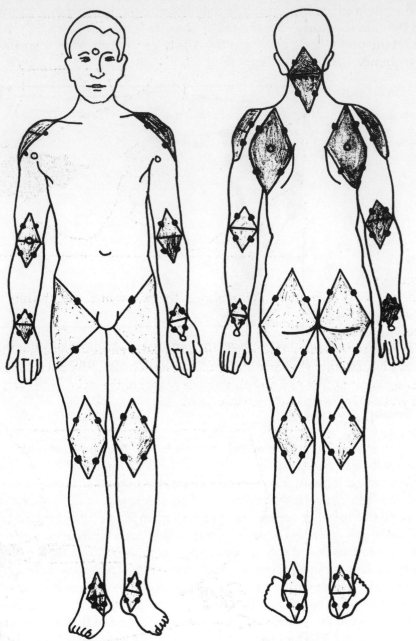

Fig. 53

Client is on his back

Step 1. Stand at the client's feet.

   2. Place your right thumb on the sole of the right foot, and your left fire finger on one of the points in the diamond-shaped pattern covering the right ankle (Fig. 54).

   3. Hold each contact area for about 1 minute until you can feel the energy strongly in the fire finger.

   4. Move the fire finger to a point beneath the right knee in the next diamond shape, and move the thumb to the position that the fire finger has just left (Fig. 55).

78

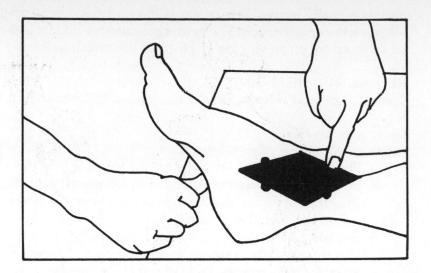

Fig. 54

5. Repeat step 3.
6. Move the fire finger to a point above the knee and the thumb to the point below it.
7. Repeat step 3.
8. Continue in this fashion until you have moved the energy above the hip joint of the right leg. Repeat steps 1 to 8 on the left leg and each arm. When working the arms the first contact point with the thumb is in the centre of the palm. You can also push the energy back down through the jaw joint.

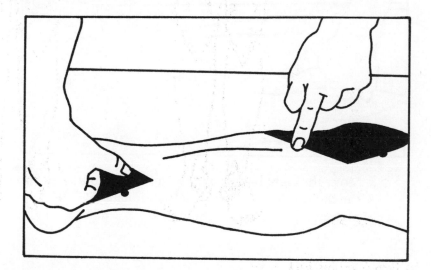

Fig. 55

Origins and Insertions Technique

This is a technique for releasing energy blocks in muscles that are manifesting as a disturbance of motor function or movement. The origin of a muscle is its point of attachment to the skeletal structure, and the insertion is the point of attachment to the bone which the muscle actually moves. The origin is the positive pole of an individual muscle and the insertion the negative pole. The neuter pole is in the middle of the muscle. Energy blocks can be released by polarising the origin with the insertion (or the neuter pole).

RELEASING THE LEG MUSCLES
This is a general release for the numerous different muscles in the upper and lower leg.

Client is on his back

Step1. Stand on the client's left side.

    2. Place your right hand underneath the left knee from the inside of the leg. You should be able to feel numerous tendons underneath your fingers. Wrap your left hand over the left foot so that the tips of your fingers press in to the tendons around the ball of the foot (Fig. 56).

    3. Stimulate alternately by pressing your fingers in to the ball of the foot, extending the toes rhythmically as you do so and using a circular movement under the back of the knee, for 2-3 minutes. Hold and feel for energy.

    4. The left hand can also move to the achilles tendon area for a more specific release of the muscles in the calf, such as the gastrocnemius muscle.

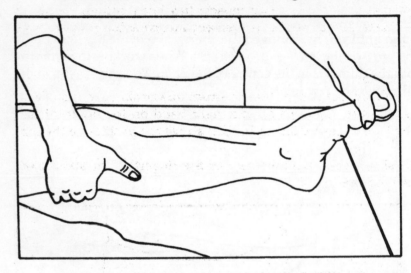

Fig. 56

    5. Move the right hand up to the tendons around the hip joint and the lower spine of the ilium (Fig. 57). Alternately stimulate this area with a circular movement as you manipulate the ball of the foot for 2-3 minutes. Hold and feel for the energy.

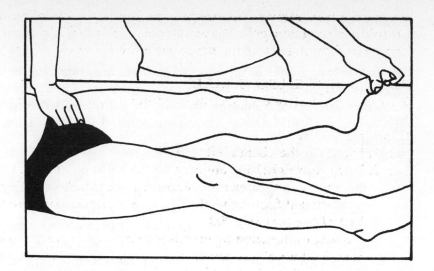

Fig. 57

RELEASING THE RECTUS FEMORIS MUSCLE

The rectus femoris muscle is one of the quadriceps muscles in the upper leg responsible for extending the knee and straightening the leg. This muscle has been chosen simply to illustrate the basic technique. The technique can be used on any muscle as long as you know the location of its origin and insertion.

Client is on his back

Step1. Stand on the client's left side.

    2. Place the fingertips of your left hand on the tendon structure just above the patella in the middle of the leg, and the fingertips of your right hand on the origin of the muscle which is on the lower anterior iliac spine just above the position of the hip joint (Fig. 58).

    3. Stimulate alternately using a circular movement of the fingertips for about two minutes. Hold and feel for energy.

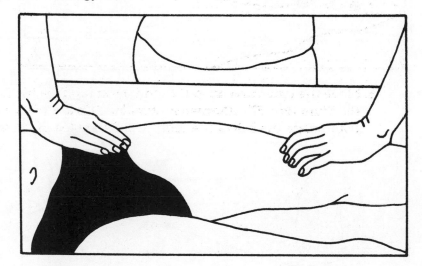

Fig. 58

Treating Pain in the Long Bones of the Legs

Pain in the long bones of the legs can indicate anaemia, lymphatic stasis, or lack of various nutrients such as vitamin C, sodium, manganese or calcium. It may also be due to exhaustion through excessive standing or walking. In many cases the roots of the pain lie in poor digestion, and should be treated with this in mind. Local release work as set out below is also applicable.

Client is on his back

Step 1. Stand on his left side.

2. Reach across his body, place your right hand on the inside of his right upper thigh and the left hand on his right lower leg (Fig. 59).

3. Grip the muscles and tendons of his inner thigh and rotate your hand in an outward direction, at the same time as you grip the muscles of the lower leg and twist the tissues inwards. Vibrate your hands for about 30 seconds. Rest for a moment, then repeat once or twice more.

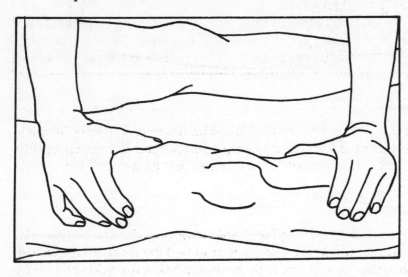

Fig. 59

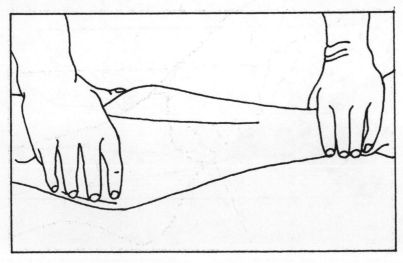

Fig. 60

4. Make other similar twisting contacts with your hands on different parts of the leg. Both contacts on the lower leg (Fig. 60) or the upper leg.
5. Finally connect an outward twisting contact on the upper (or lower leg) to a contact on the pelvis. The pelvic contact can be done either with an upward vibration or a rocking movement (Fig. 61).

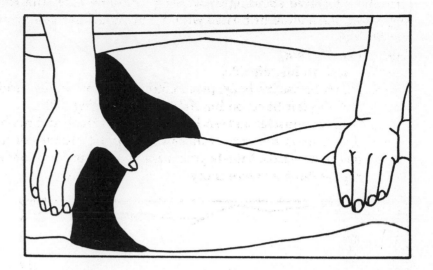

Fig. 61

Correction for a Low Arch

This technique is a correction for a client who has collapsed arches in one or both feet. It is important that the arches of the feet are structured appropriately. Correcting the arches can release many reflexes to the body and eliminate a lot of aches and pains due to structural imbalance.

Client is on his back

Step 1. Stand at the client's feet.

2. To treat the right foot, grip the arch of the foot firmly with your right hand (Fig. 62), and with your left hand grip the outside of the foot so that the fingers support the heel and the palm covers the cuboid bone with the thumb below the ankle bone (Fig. 63).

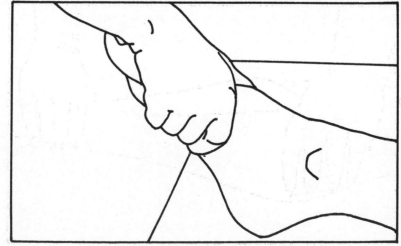

Fig. 62

3. Hold each contact firmly until you can feel the energy flowing strongly, and then the arch correction is a simultaneous twist of the right hand and a quick short thrust of the left hand to the right. See directional arrows in Fig. 63.

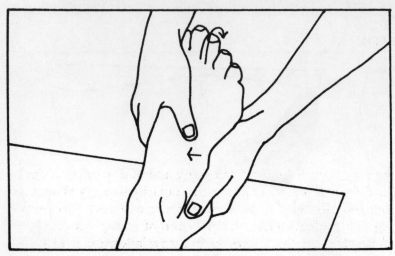

Fig. 63

8.   Structural Balancing

Structural balancing refers to the aspect of the energy-balancing and bodywork that deals specifically with balancing the body's relationship to gravity. In polarity therapy balancing the body's relationship with gravity is considered to be the final phase of the whole energy-balancing process. It is the phase that deals with the crystallisation of energy into form or matter, the physical body. Structural balancing deals with the body's relationship to external forces, in particular the force of gravity as the predominating external force acting on the body throughout its lifetime.

The crystallisation process that forms the physical structure occurs in much the same way a saline solution will form salt crystals if left over a period of time. In the human being this crystallisation into form is governed by the energy body, the organising matrix. The solution from which the body is formed is the five primordial elements. The fundamental structure is formed in the womb. The environment within the womb is an external factor that can profoundly influence the basic structure. Even should no structural distortion occur pre-birth, it will almost certainly begin under the influence of all the various external factors that act from the moment of birth. Physical growth continues up to about twenty-five years of age and it is during this period that the structure tends to deform most, to literally lose its original form. From birth, gravity and air pressure are the first forces that act upon the organism. Gravity is the most intense of the primary acting forces and it continues to act throughout life as a de-forming stress.

Whilst the metaphor of 'crystallisation' is useful in describing the process of creation, it is less useful when it comes to trying to elucidate the dynamic process that is 'life'. The human body is in actual fact an amazingly plastic, malleable system. You have only to compare a photograph of yourself taken today with one taken ten or twenty years ago to realise the truth of that statement.

Gravity is the major external force acting on the body. It is not the only one, but because it is the major one, the way in which the body and self deals with it is a metaphor for the way in which all other external forces are dealt with. Most of the energy-balancing in polarity therapy deals with inner relationships, e.g. the relationship between the self, the emotions and the vital physiological functioning. Structural balancing deals with outer relationships, e.g. the body's relationship with gravity, but also in a much broader sense with the life as a whole; human relationships; work; leisure activities and so on. The way a client organises themselves in relation to gravity tells a great deal about the way in which they deal with life. The degree to which a client's body distorts in relation to gravity also tells you the degree to which they distort in relation to all other external factors. It is my opinion that the impact of

85

intimate personal relationships can be considered as the next major force acting on us after gravity. Much can be learned from the gravity board concerning the way a client deals with personal relationships. When a client is lying on the table they are in a sense off gravity, it is no longer acting on their structure in the same way, so what you are seeing is in effect more of their relationship to their inner forces, their vital energies and functioning (see Chapter 3). You could say that there are two different kinds of body reading: one done in relation to gravity and one not. Body reading done in relation to gravity tells you about a client's relationship with their outer life; how they deal with external forces and other people. Body reading done when the body is off gravity tells you about the client's relationship with their inner life, how they deal with their thoughts and feelings about themselves. As a polarity therapist it can provide invaluable information concerning the true nature of the client's problems to read the body in both ways and to correlate both.

It is important to realise that a client can be, to use Dr. Stone's words, 'humpbacked and all distorted, yet live to a ripe old age'. It is not structural distortions that kill us but the cessation of our vital physiological functioning. All organs within the body need sufficient room to expand and contract, and should the structure be causing such a lack of space then it is obviously creating a very real health problem. However, correcting the outer structure does not necessarily mean that you are going to be correcting impaired physiological functioning. Reading the body in relation to gravity tells a great deal about structural distortions and the body's ability to adapt to stress, but tells nothing about the status of the internal physiological and energetic functions. It is possible for a client to have a well balanced structure in relation to gravity and yet still have severe internal disturbances. The key factor to remember is that the life energy is beyond the influence of gravity, and so the body's relationship to gravity is not a useful guide to the health of the client. Dr. Stone points out that it is more a guide to the capacity for movement and the relationship of parts.

What is the relationship between the energy and the structure? The first point to understand is that it is the muscles that determine the boney alignment of the structure; to be specific, the balance of muscular tension between the various groups of muscles. It is obvious, then, that the relationship we are looking for is that between the muscles and the life energy. The link is obviously the emotions. We all know just how profoundly our posture and therefore our muscular tension changes in relation to our state of being. Think back to the last time you felt happy and joyful, I can guarantee that you stood taller, straighter and moved far more easily than normal. What about a time when you felt depressed? I have no doubt that some combination of the following things occurred: your diaphragm tensed up, your breathing became shallow and as a consequence your lumbar curve increased giving you quite a sway back; your shoulders slumped, your neck collapsed and so on. Any disturbance to the free flow of emotion can result in a pattern of muscular tension that is often referred to as body 'armouring'. Emotional disturbances and their related patterns of muscular armouring make it impossible for the body to adapt in an efficient way to the external force of gravity. This relationship of energy to structure is in the step down or involutionary phase of energy movement, during which consciousness and energy manifest into physical form.

If the flow of life energy can influence the structure in a dynamic way throughout life, what, if any, influence does the structure have on the energy? On the basis of what Dr. Stone said, as quoted earlier, it would seem that he felt the structure had very little influence on the flow of life energy. However, in other places he does set out a certain level of influence that structural distortion created through external environmental factors has on vital functioning.

Leaving aside such situations as physical trauma caused by accident or surgical operation, perhaps the major source of structural distortions is from the actions we do habitually over long periods of time in the course of our daily lives as we work and play. For example, suppose you have a client who is a farmer who spends many hours driving a tractor, looking backwards over his left shoulder with his body twisted so that he can watch what he is doing. Over the years he will have developed a major distortion of the muscular tension patterns in his body, to the point where it will need only a small amount of extra stress to cause a structural collapse. He has come to you after months of varying degrees of pain, and the one thing that you can be sure of is that he is going to have severe diaphragmatic spasm, and that same spasm which will have been there since the initial collapse will by now be interfering in the flow of many different patterns of energy in the body, with such attendant problems as poor digestion, suppressed breathing and constipation. The thing to remember is that, as in our earlier discussion of armouring, any painful structural disturbance will create an emotional disturbance, so ultimately the internal process is similar. The main factor here is time. We know that an effective energy-balancing manipulation, which can be done in a few moments, can sometimes change the structure instantly, because energy is the organising factor of the physical form as an entropic or step-down process; the reverse reaction, however, requires a great deal of energy. The physical structure, which is basically energy vibrating at a very low frequency, has to apply that energy over a long period of time to be able to influence higher frequencies to any great degree.

In structural balancing you are re-structuring the body in relation to gravity, so that you have a symmetrically balanced posture which is vertical or at a perfect right-angle to its base on the earth (the soles of the feet): see Fig. 64. This particular postural orientation is indicative of a perfect balance of both inner and outer forces. However, it should be borne in mind that few people actually have the kind of symmetrically balanced bone structure that would allow a perfect relationship to gravity. When re-checking a client's alignment after a structural session, do not get too attached to seeing a client exhibit the perfect structure, as shown here.

The body reading that is part of structural balancing is done on the gravity board. It uses a plumb line as the guide to the way a body should organise itself in relation to gravity if it is to be considered to be economically working with the force rather than against it. The plumb line is also the mirror that shows precisely how the body is deforming in relation to gravity. When a client is standing on the gravity board, what you see are the distortions of the skeletal frame caused by unequal muscular tensions. There are many different lines of stress in the physical body that relate to the force of gravity (see Fig. 65). An understanding of these patterns and the dynamic way that the body compensates when any such stress lines become distorted is essential to your ability to rebalance the structure.

Figs 66 and 67 show some important structural relationships in the body. Fig. 66 shows the energy pattern known as the interlaced triangles or six-pointed star (Seal of Solomon). This representation of the six-pointed star differs slightly from the classical structure, but Dr. Stone says that it is the correct orientation of the structure within the human body. Esoterically, this symbol represents a meeting of heaven and earth. The inverted triangle represents the creation of matter from spirit, the masculine principle; and the other triangle pointing upwards represents man's return path to heaven, the feminine principle. The interlacing of the two triangles is indicative of perfect balance between these two principles. Structurally the chart shows, when looking at the back of the body, that the base of the lower triangle cuts through the sacro-iliac articulations and the apex touches the area of the brain

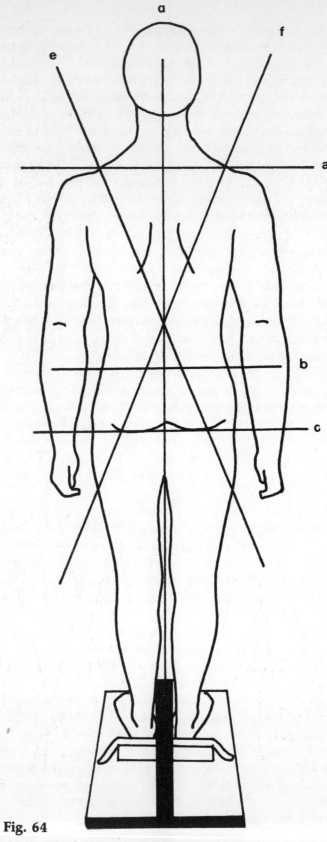

Fig. 64

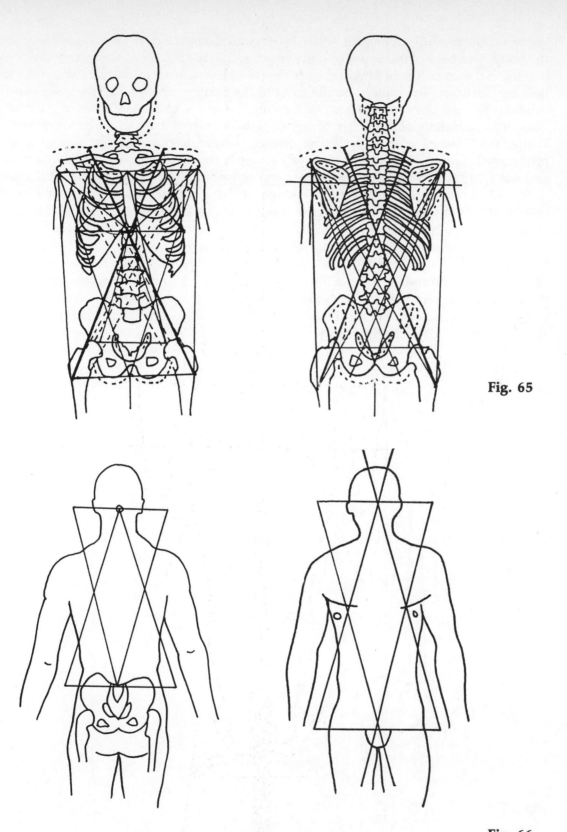

Fig. 65

Fig. 66

known as the medulla oblongata, which is the central control for the autonomic functions in the body. The base of the upper triangle cuts through the foramen magnum of the occipital bone and the apex touches into the very centre of the sacrum, midway between the sacro-iliac articulations. The pattern on the front of the body covers a slightly broader area; the orbital ridge and the symphysis pubis forming the upper and lower bases of the triangles. This shows a linking of the centre of consciousness or third eye and the generative organs. Whilst the balance of this particular energy pattern is obviously important from the physiological point of view, it also indicates the structural relationship between the sacrum and the occiput as well as in a more general sense the head's relationship to the pelvis.

Fig. 67 shows some further relationships of the head, neck and pelvis. It shows the relationship between the occiput and the sacrum as being a diamond or kite shaped structure of two triangles, the upper triangle being the occiput and the lower triangle the sacrum. Dr. Stone talked of a gyroscopic balance occurring between these two bones. The lines in the figure marked 'a' show the relationship between the middle of the shoulder, sacral apex and sacro-iliac articulation on each side. Line 'b' shows the relationship between the mandibular joint with the hip joint, as well as the temporal bone with the innominate bone. Line 'c' is indicative of the relationship between the occipital base and the sacral base, which should both be horizontal.

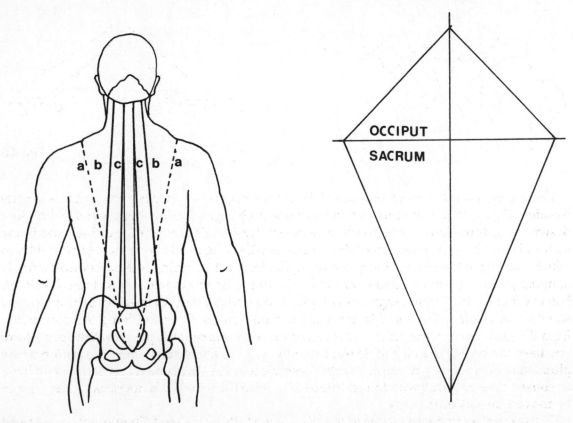

Fig. 67

90

The energy pattern of the five pointed star, or pentagram, when superimposed on the human body, shows the relationship between the hips and shoulders as diagonal lines of energy or stress. It also shows a vertical relationship between the hip joints as the foundation to the occiput, and the position of the head generally. This pattern has been dealt with in some detail elsewhere so I do not propose to deal with it in any greater depth here, other than to indicate its relevance to structural work.

Fig. 68 shows the architectural structure of the relationship between the sacrum and the hip joints as being a cantilever. In a structurally balanced body the whole weight of the upper body structure falls directly down into the sacrum, which then properly stresses the pelvic structure as a keystone in a bridge. The cantilever structure is the thick posterior arch structure of the pelvis, which is formed by the three upper sacral vertebrae as its keystone and the thick bone structure of the lower part of the ilium as its sides. The cantilever is anchored to the head of the femur by the ilio-femoral ligament. This particular set-up allows the weight of the upper body to be supported without any muscular effort, because the downward force at the sacral end of the cantilever is held in check by the fixed ends of the cantilever at the head of the femurs. It is only when the pelvis is functioning in this way that you can have a truly light and lively walking action.

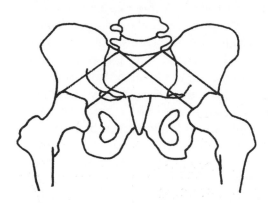 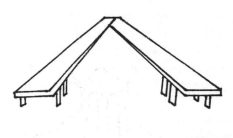

Fig. 68

The gravity board is made of a board 24 inches long by 12 inches wide. It has a central wooden divider that is 2½ inches wide and one inch high. This divider should have a line drawn along its full length which is in the exact centre line. The cross piece or backstop is one inch wide and 2 inches high. There should be a small spring fixed to one end of the divider to which you attach the plumb line when using the board. The spring is used because a freely hanging plumb bob moves about far too easily. In the first instance, you will need a plumb bob to establish the correct alignment of board and string. Later, for speed of setting up, you should always place the board in the same position on the floor and hang the plumb line from the same spot on the ceiling. This can be done by marking the place on the floor where you have the board, so that you do not have always to re-check its position in relation to the plumb line every time you use it. It is also possible to do as Dr. Stone recommends and have the board close to a wall with hinges attached to it, so that when it is not in use it can simply be moved up out of the way.

To use the gravity board you need the client to be fully undressed. They stand on the front half of the board so that their heels fit snugly into the backstop of the central divider on the board, the insides of the feet touching the central divider. Get them to focus their eyes on a point on the wall at eye level as this helps to prevent undue swaying of the body. Sit behind them and take a line of sight which always keeps the plumb line aligned with the centre line of the board. Having studied their positioning for a few moments to gain an overall sense of their structural relationship, take a skin pencil or felt-tip pen and mark any tense muscles which are bulging towards you with a plus sign and any hollow areas with a minus sign. This is important because when the client lies down the tension patterns are often changed or reversed. It is a reminder to you of where you need to work. These areas marked plus and minus can be polarised with each other or to the centre of gravity of the body. In Fig. 64 you will see a body that is lining up perfectly with gravity. The upper horizontal line marked 'a' shows level shoulders. The horizontal line marked 'b' shows level innominate bones. The horizontal line marked 'c' shows a level sacral base. The central vertical line (the plumb line) marked 'd' shows a perfectly straight spine with no rotation. Note also that the shoulder blades are level and that there are no skin folds showing in the waist area. The diagonal lines marked 'e' and 'f' are a diagonal or five-pointed star relationship of lines of stress that pass from the hips through the sacro-iliac articulations to the middle points of each shoulder. These two lines cross between the second and third lumbar vertebrae which is at the same level as the umbilicus. Dr. Stone points out that this is the centre of gravity in the body. This is an ideal body pattern which is the ultimate goal of structural balancing.

When looking at a new client on the gravity board for the first time, I begin my reading from the bottom up, beginning with checking line 'c' beneath the buttocks. I normally make a diagrammatic sketch of my findings as I go along. I then check to see whether the plumb line falls directly between the crease in the buttocks. If it falls either to the left or the right it indicates a body rotation to that side. I then check line 'b', for the hip level. At this point I look at the spinal alignment against the plumb line to see whether there is any scoliosis or curvature, and note this. I note any skin folds in the waist area caused by contracted muscle groupings on one side or the other. Finally, I note the high shoulder, indicated by line 'a' (the crease at the arm pit is another useful indicator of shoulder height), the scapula position by looking at the bone structure, and lastly the orientation of the head. I also check the degree of lordosis (lumbar curvature) in the lower back by taking a side view.

It is important to remember that the gravity board is no kind of indicator of the client's state of health. If a client is complaining of severe lower back pains and yet lines up straight and level on the gravity board, then, as Dr. Stone points out, you are probably dealing with prostatic trouble if it is a male client or uterine disturbance in a female. Please bear in mind that structurally corrective techniques are *not* given when there is acute pain. It is vital to get rid of the pain first through releasing the energy blocks before trying to make structural corrections. Indeed, getting rid of the energy blocks is often all that is required, as the structure sorts itself out through the action of the sympathetic nervous system.

Before looking in more detail at the kind of structural distortions you may see when using the gravity board I want to discuss my basic approach to the practice and teaching of structural balancing. The first point I want to make is that in no way can structural balancing be taught as a science. By this, I mean that you cannot look at a body and say the client has a left short leg due to an inferior anterior sacral base on that side, plus high left shoulder and a posteriority of the left innominate, and treat it by techniques A, B and C. The body does not react in that way nor are the effects of the techniques so predictable, due to the dynamic and individual way each person compensates for their various adaptations to gravity. The approach I use is one of playing with and through the structure of the body, doing a small amount of work and then checking the effect on the gravity board so that I begin to get a

Fig. 69

Fig. 70

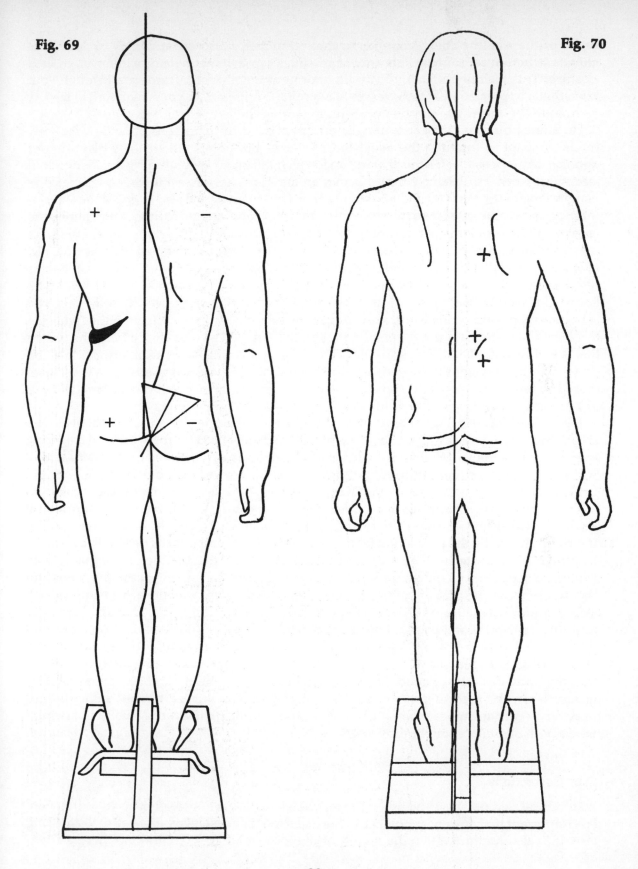

sense of the way the client responds to the techniques. I also use my body to mimic the client's structure as an immediate way of gaining a sense of the dynamics involved in their posture. This technique can give you an enormous amount of information through your kinesthetic appreciation of the stresses and strains this creates in your own body. Like any technique the more you practise postural mirroring the better you become.

Dr. Stone points out a few common distortions of the body in his books, and how the body tends to adapt as found in the usual run of clients, but points out that *any* distortion or abnormality is possible. It is this that makes it really difficult to generalise when talking about structural work. For example, he says that an anterior inferior sacral base on either side usually creates the short leg and low shoulder on the same side. He also says that the anterior inferior sacral base side is also the side of the body that moves anterior unless, and here is the essence of the problem, there are other complicating twists and distortions or where over a period of time the natural compensatory function of the body has changed the situation. Fig. 69 shows the typical result of a tilt of the sacral base as described above. The sacral base is tilted to the right, creating a low right shoulder and a general contraction on that side of the body. The sacral position is indicated by the right buttock being lower than the left. The actual sacral position shown is greatly exaggerated for clarity. In this situation the right side of the body is often anterior (a rotation to the right), as indicated by the fact that the plumb line is falling to the left of the centre line. The minus signs will show the anterior side of the body, and the plus signs the posterior side. In clients who have excess body fat at waist level there is often a crease on the opposite side of the body to that in which the sacrum is tilting; in this case the skin crease or fold is on the left side.

Fig. 70 is a drawing of a photograph of the structural alignment of an actual client as they stood on the gravity board. This same client was the model used for the structural balancing treatments that follow. Whilst it has not been written up as an illustrated case history study I will make some comments throughout on the kind of changes that took place, as well as a more detailed look at the end on the overall changes that took place over three sessions of structural bodywork. Looking back to the figure the first thing to note from the buttock level line is that the sacral base was inferior and anterior on the right side. The body was rotated to the right, shown by the plumb line falling to the left of the centre line. The left iliac crest is a little high. Note the tension in the left gluteal muscles. The right shoulder is dropped, which is most noticeable from the crease at the armpit rather than the top line of the shoulders and the difference in the position of the scapula. Note the different way the arms hang on each side of the body and the breadth of the upper body relative to the pelvis. There is also a lot of muscular tension near the right shoulder and in the lumbar area on both sides (marked with plus signs). Lastly the plumb line indicated no spinal compensation for the sacral position and the head is also in line with the spine. This last fact is most interesting because it means that his body has a layer of adaptation overlaid on top of the natural compensation that occurs when the sacrum is out of position. The client had injured himself some months previously carrying a heavy weight, and was experiencing quite a lot of pain in the sacrum when both stationary and in movement.

Foot Corrections

A structural session always begins at the feet, as a structure is only as good as its foundation. It is important that any energy blocks in the feet should be resolved before you do anything else. It is also important that the arches of the foot are in good condition. There are two

94

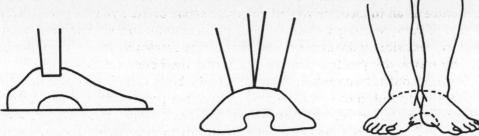

Fig. 71

arches in the foot, the longitudinal and the transverse. The longitudinal arch is shown on the left of Fig. 71 and the transverse in the middle. On the right it shows how the transverse arch of each foot forms a complete structure when taken together. The leg pull in the general energy-balancing session is a correction for a high arch, and the correction for a low arch or flat foot is shown on page 83.

OS CALCIS CORRECTION

The os calcis bone or calcaneum is the foundation bone of the body structure. It is the negative pole of the occiput, the sacrum being the neuter pole. There is very often tenderness around the heel on the short leg side and severe occipital tension, though

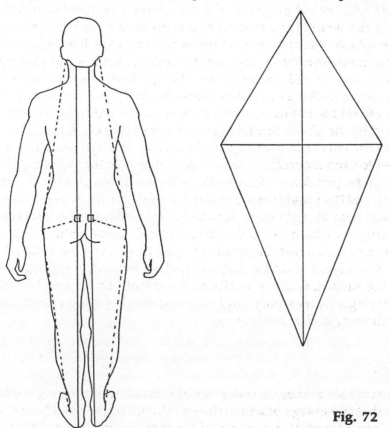

Fig. 72

95

occasionally the occipital tension manifests on the opposite side. It is usually the heel bone on the short leg side that is most distorted, and so the technique is usually done on the short leg side. However, both ankles can be out of line in which case both are treated. Fig. 72 shows as a straight line the pull of gravity from the heel bones through the sacro-iliac articulation to the occiput, and as dotted lines the energy waves radiating from the occiput down through the muscles of the back through the hip joints to the heels. The integrity of these lines of energy determines the posture in relation to gravity. The left side of Fig. 72 shows the relationship between the force of gravity and the energy waves as being like the rigging of a ship's mast, which is the only way to stabilise a tall structure like the body. The os calcis correction has a great deal of effect on body rotation, and bodily rotation is one of the main indicators for its usage. Remember the body frequently rotates to the inferior anterior sacral base side.

Normal heel positioning allows free movement of the ankle in either direction (Fig. 73). A typical distortion is seen in Fig. 74 and this is also the actual position of the os calcis bone of our client. It is the heel of the short leg side that is the most distorted.

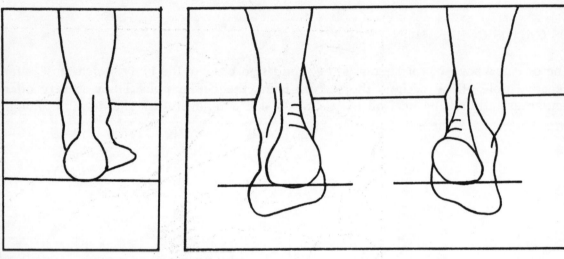

Fig. 73　　　**Fig. 74**

Client is on his front

Step 1. Stand on his right side.

2. Raise the right foot, and with your right thumb contact the sorest point just above the heel on the outside of the os calcis bone. The fingers are placed over the heel base so that the tips rest on the inside of the heel.

3. Contact the diaphragm reflex area on the foot with the thumb of your left hand (Fig 75).

4. Alternately stimulate the diaphragm reflex with a circular movement while holding the heel bone in an outwards direction, maintaining the thumb pressure on the sore spot. Do this for 1-2 minutes until you can feel the energy strongly.

5. Lay the leg down and make the same corrective heel contact but this time with the left hand, and with the right hand rock the client's right thigh in the same direction (in particular any tense muscle groups). Stimulate for 1-2 minutes until you can feel the energy flowing.

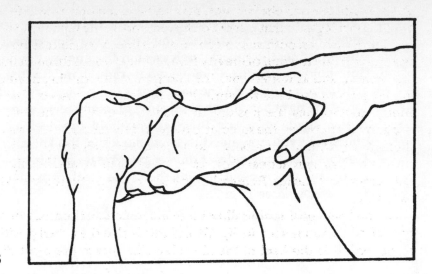

Fig. 75

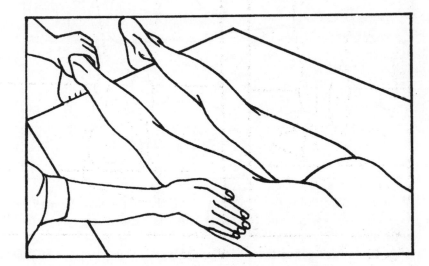

Fig. 76

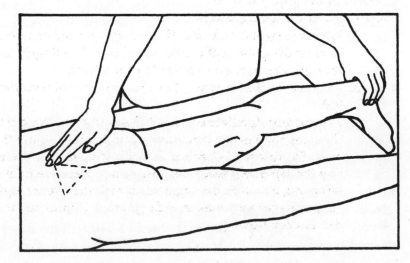

Fig. 77

6. Keeping the same heel contact, move the right hand up to the hip joint and contact any tight muscles around the joint with your fingertips. Stimulate for 1-2 minutes until you feel the muscles release and the energy flowing strongly (Fig. 76).
7. Still holding the heel, move your right hand to the client's right sacro-iliac articulation. Stimulate the sacral joint for 1-2 minutes (Fig. 77).
8. Move the right hand up the body to contact any tense areas on the back (marked with a plus sign). Stimulate them as you hold the heel for 1-2 minutes. To do this effectively you may need to bend the leg at the knee.
9. Contact the sorest side of the occipital ridge. In this case it is the client's left side. Stimulate the occiput as you hold the heel contact for 1-2 minutes until the tenderness eases (Fig. 78).

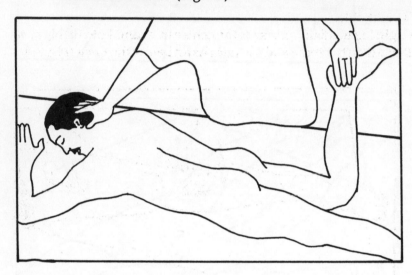

Fig. 78

If the client's heel is twisting outwards the sore spot to work on is on the inside of the heel. The correction, no matter what the distortion, is always to level the heel base and re-align it.

At this point place the client's feet back on the bolster or just over the edge of the couch and you should find the heels are level. Ask him to stand on the gravity board so you can see how this has changed the overall structure. I have had clients whose *whole* structure has re-aligned after one os calcis treatment! In this particular case the rotation vanished but little else changed.

Short Leg Corrections

The short leg side is caused by sacral distortion and muscular imbalance in the pelvis. It is indicative of an overall contraction in the energy currents on that side of the body. Dr. Stone said that when the short leg side lengthens and stays long, normal repair processes are able to take place within the body. It would also indicate that the sacrum was level and that the muscular and energetic forces around it are balanced. There are various techniques that release the short side and they can be done independently of a full structural balancing session. A short leg correction as a specific treatment need not be done during a structural session as any sacral correction will always correct the short leg. However, the treatment given below is a valuable release to use as you work up the body during a structural balancing session.

SHORT LEG RELEASE BY TORQUE

The short leg side is often the tense leg side. To determine the short and tense leg have the client on their back and with your air fingers simultaneously push each foot towards the centre line of the body (medial rotation) and compare the tension and resistance to movement. The leg that is most difficult to move is the short and tense leg.

Returning to our client whose short and tense leg is the right:

Client is on his back
Step 1. Stand on the client's right side.
   2. Pick up and rotate the right leg medially (towards the centre line) and hold in this position by having the left hand on the thigh and the right hand below the knee (Fig. 79).

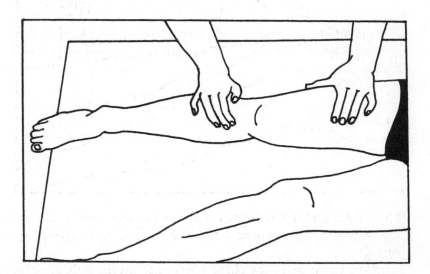

Fig. 79

   3. Holding the leg in this position, rock it gently and rhythmically towards the centre line. The whole body should begin to rock gently. Continue rocking for 2-3 minutes until the muscles release. The hand positions can be changed during the treatment, moving up and down the leg but still keeping it medially rotated. It is particularly beneficial to release the thigh muscles in relation to the anterior pelvic muscles, still rocking the leg inwards (see Fig. 80).

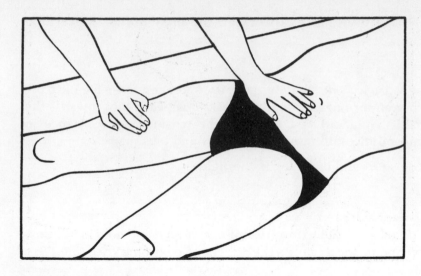

Fig. 80

Sacral Corrections

Dr. Stone called the sacrum the key to the body structure and function. It is the focal point where all the physical stresses and strains and the force of gravity meet in the body. The relationship between the sacrum and the head of the femur via the muscular attachments is of paramount importance in maintaining the upright posture of the body. The relationship between the sacrum and the other bones of the pelvis is no less important. The sacrum moves very little within the pelvis, it is bound very strongly in place by various ligaments. The sacro-iliac articulation limits the movement of the sacrum to a slight gliding rotation between the sacrum and the posterior portion of the ilium. The actual amount of movement we are talking about is a few millimetres only. However, the degree of muscular pull needed to move the sacrum out of its natural position and maintain that distortion is enormous. A look at the actual boney structure of the pelvis will show you that when we talk of the sacrum as moving posterior that does not literally mean that it has moved behind the restraint of the ilium. To do so would actually require many centimetres of movement to take place. When we say that one of the corners of the sacral base has moved posterior it means that it is posterior in relation to the other side of the sacral base, which has actually moved a few millimetres anteriorly within the pelvis. This kind of posterior-anterior movement by the sacrum is nearly always accompanied by a downwards slippage or tilting of the sacrum towards the side that has moved anteriorly.

In actual practice before trying to rebalance or reposition the sacrum it is important to release the deep interior muscle spasm that is holding the sacrum in position. This is usually best accomplished by giving the client a perineal treatment and polarising the perineal contact with the related sore points in the neck, the shoulders and the sorest spot in the back. It is also useful to balance tenderness in the buttocks with tender areas on and around the shoulder blades (as per Fig. 46 page 72). A five-pointed star release on the front of the body as a final relaxation of the psoas and iliacus muscles may also be valuable.

Returning now to our client whose sacrum is anterior and inferior on the right side:

TECHNIQUE 1
Client is on his front
Step 1. Stand on the client's left side.

100

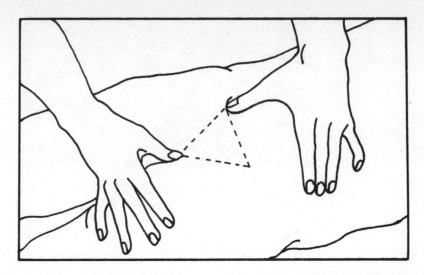

Fig. 81

2. With your left thumb contact the left side of the sacral base, the thumb pointing downwards. With your right thumb contact the apex of the sacrum, the thumb pointing diagonally towards the right hip (Fig. 81).
3. The position of the thumbs indicates the direction of vibratory impulses to be applied to the sacrum. Vibrate gently for 1-2 minutes.
4. Position the thumbs as in Fig. 82 and vibrate directionally for 1-2 minutes.
5. Place the right hand over the sacrum, the fingers pointing towards the right side, and the left hand on the positive pole of the sacrum, the occipital bone (Fig. 83). Rotate the right hand anti-clockwise some 20 degrees. Apply a gentle vibration with the right hand giving the sacrum a corrective directional impulse downwards and anterior through the heel of the palm for one minute. Feel for an energetic balance in both hands.

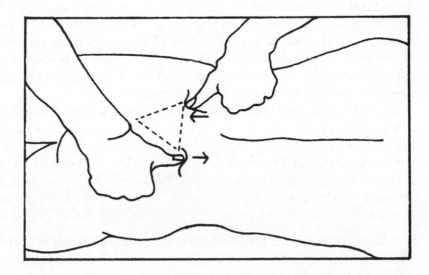

Fig. 82

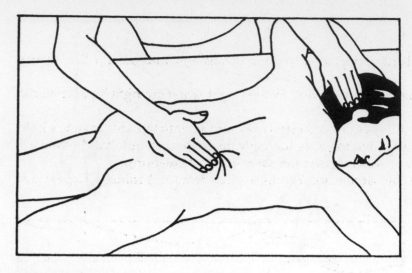

Fig. 83

TECHNIQUE 2
Client is on his front
Step 1. Stand on client's left side.
    2. Place the right fire finger on the apex of the sacrum, palm up, and place the left fire finger on the spine of the ilium near the left sacro-iliac joint (Fig. 84).

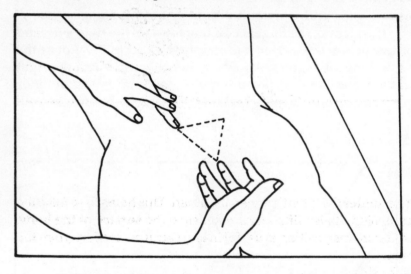

Fig. 84

3. The left fire finger is held steady, whilst the right fire finger gives a movement that is directed towards the head and is also lightly lifting the apex of the sacrum posteriorly. You are trying to bring the sacrum back into a balanced position. The palm-up position of the right hand helps to remind you that the impulse on the sacrum is not anterior, which would only tend to increase the distortion. The vibratory, directional impulse is given for 1-2 minutes.

4. Leave the right fire finger in place on the apex of the sacrum, and place the left hand on the occipital area of the head as in step 5 of technique 1. Holding the upper contact still, vibrate the sacral contact gently upwards toward the head for approximately one minute. Then hold both areas and feel for an energetic balance.

TECHNIQUE 3

Client is on his left side.

Step 1. Stand behind the client and place a bolster or cushion underneath the client's left hip.

2. Contact the apex of the sacrum with the left fire finger while the right hand is on the iliac crest (Fig. 85).

3. Gently vibrate and lift the apex of the sacrum towards the right hip, as you gently hold the iliac crest in an upward and towards-the-table position (this right-hand action is a slight rolling movement which opens the sacro-iliac articulation).

4. Stimulate the apex of the sacrum for 1 minute, then rest for 1 minute. Repeat this sequence 4 or 5 times.

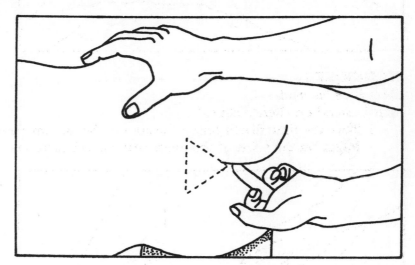

Fig. 85

TECHNIQUE 4

Client is on his front

Step 1. Place a bolster or cushion under the client's lower abdomen. This helps to release the sacral lock and lumbar tension. It also lifts sacral reflexes to the surface of the body. The placement of a cushion in this position is useful in any sacral correction when the client is lying face down.

2. Stand at the client's right side.

3. With your left arm bend the client's legs until they are at right-angles to the table. With the thumb of the right hand support the right side of the sacral triangle in an upward direction towards the left hip.

4. Supporting the sacrum, rock the client's legs towards you for 1-2 minutes. If his flexibility will allow, you may also fold the calves closer to the thighs than is shown (Fig. 86).

5. The thumb contact with the right hand may be changed to a heel-of-the-palm contact (Fig. 87). This contact can be used all the way up the back on tense spinal muscles as well. This is a powerful technique — be very sensitive to any discomfort that it may cause the client.

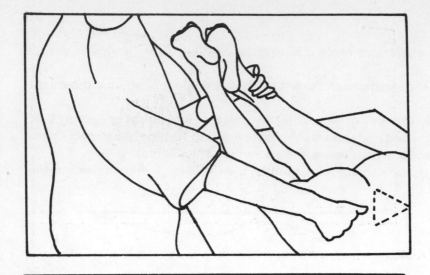

Fig. 86

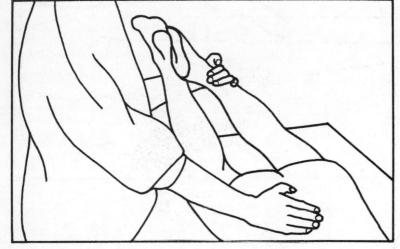

Fig. 87

TECHNIQUE 5

This technique is a manipulation of the interlaced triangles (Fig. 66), and as such will influence much more than the sacral position. It is useful in cases of bladder trouble, menstrual disorders, leg cramps and is also an excellent release for the sinuses.

Client is on his back

Step 1. Stand at the client's left side.

   2. Place your left hand over the left-hand side of the client's symphysis pubis, and the thumb of your right hand on the right side of the pubis.

   3. Using a rocking action, the left hand is moved in an upwards direction whilst the thumb of the right hand works downwards into the contracted muscle tissues next to the bone, working all the way along the right side of the pubis. The angle of application of your contacts may be varied to facilitate the best possible release (Fig. 88).

Note: The illustrations opposite are a view of this technique from the right side of the client.

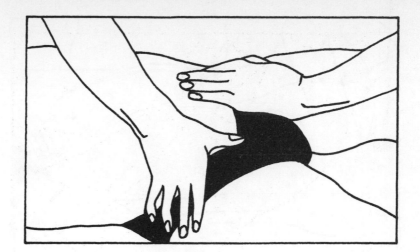

Fig. 88

4. Finally a moulding rocking release may be done using both hands (Fig. 89).

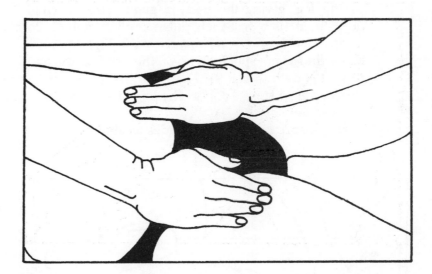

Fig. 89

Hip Correction

Having re-positioned the sacrum, you need to balance the relationship between the hip joint and the pelvis. The technique that follows is not just a hip correction but is a release of spastic tissue and energy. The technique is to locate sore points in the gluteal muscles, and then, taking a line from the sore point through the head of the femur, place the length of the femur along a continuation of the imaginary line that connects the two points. This gives you the line of force in giving the adjustment.

Client is on his side.

Step 1. Stand in front of the client.

    2. If you find a sore spot in the mid buttock area then lining up the sore point, head of the femur and leg will be as shown in Fig. 90.

    3. Place your left hand on the front of the left shoulder, and hold the hip with the thumb of your right hand on the head of the femur and the fingers stretched to cover the sore point.

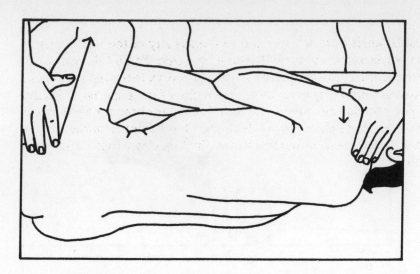

Fig. 90

4. Take up the slack in the body by pushing the shoulder back and pulling down the line of the leg, giving the body a gentle stretch. Hold for a moment and then the adjustment is a half-inch pulse applied at both contact points. The direction of application is shown by the arrows in Fig. 90.
5. If you find a sore spot high up on the buttocks the position of the leg would be similar to that shown in Fig. 91. Note that the leg is much straighter.
6. Proceed as in steps 3 and 4. The line of application is shown in Fig. 91 by directional arrows.
7. Treat all sore spots on both sides as above.

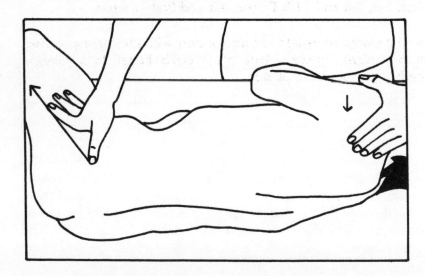

Fig. 91

Spinal Balancing

At this point in the structural balancing work you need to release any of the tense muscle fibres in the back that you have marked on the client with a plus sign. To do this you could use a variety of approaches from connecting the perineal floor or coccyx to the tense areas, to single and double hand contacts with or against the current flow (see page 64). Having released any tense muscles you should then check the individual vertebrae for tenderness and polarise them with all the other vertebrae with which they have a correspondence, as shown in Fig. 92. Other than the correspondences shown in this chart there are other correspondences set out below:

1st Dorsal — 2nd Dorsal
1st Cervical — 3rd Dorsal
2nd Cervical — 4th Dorsal
3rd Cervical — 5th Dorsal
4th Cervical — 6th Dorsal
5th Cervical — 7th Dorsal
6th Cervical — 8th Dorsal
7th Cervical — 9th Dorsal

These are structural relationships, but as Dr. Stone points out the functional effect on the physiology when sore vertebrae are balanced is just as great. The vertebrae corresponding to the various physiological systems are as follows:

Circulatory System 7th Cervical, 1st, 2nd, 9th and 10th Dorsal
Respiratory System 3rd Cervical, 3rd and 5th Dorsal, 3rd Lumbar
Digestive System 6th Cervical, 4th, 8th and 12th Dorsal, 4th Lumbar
Glandular System 4th Cervical, 3rd Dorsal, 5th Lumbar
Eliminative System 5th Cervical, 6th, 7th and 11th Dorsal, 1st and 2nd Lumbar

When balancing sore vertebrae it would be usual to balance it only with the corresponding vertebrae that are actually showing signs of distress. However, it can be beneficial to balance all the related vertebrae whether they are sore or not.

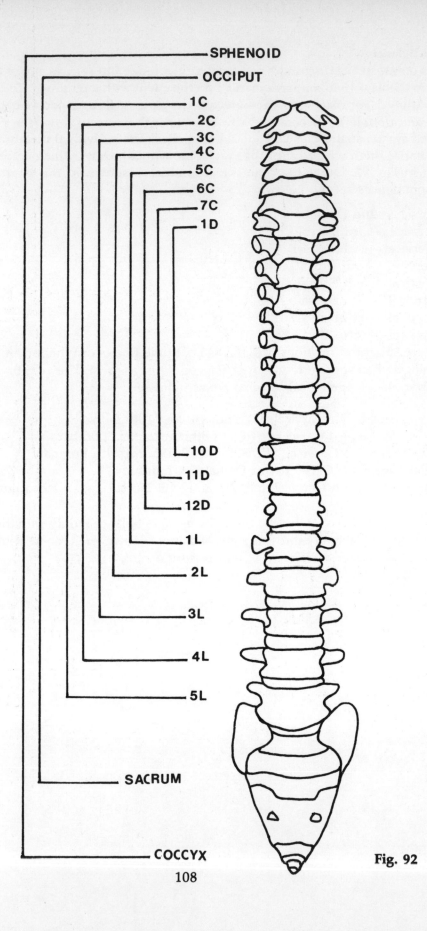

SPHENOID

OCCIPUT

1C
2C
3C
4C
5C
6C
7C
1D

10 D

11D

12D

1L

2L

3L

4L

5L

SACRUM

COCCYX

Fig. 92

108

Client is on his front

Step 1. Stand at client's left side.

2. Keeping the left hand higher on the spine, use the tips of the thumb and air fingers to contact the transverse process of the vertebrae to be balanced (Fig. 93). Alternatively, you may use the tip of the thumb and second knuckle of the air finger as contacts (Fig. 94).

3. Stimulate alternately for 1-2 minutes or longer until the tenderness is gone.

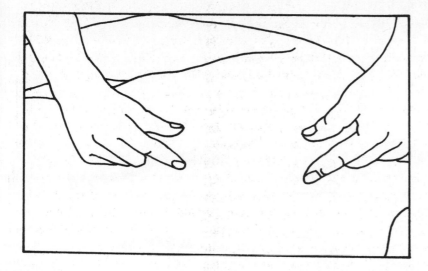

Fig. 93

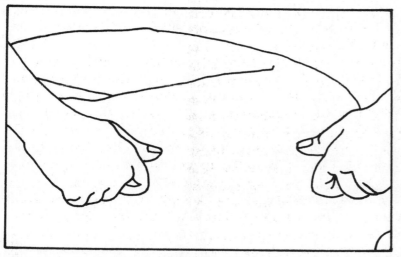

Fig. 94

Note: It is important to release the negative pole lock to any sore vertebrae by polarising it with the reflex area on the feet before working the corresponding vertebrae. The relationship between the feet and the spinal vertebrae is shown in Fig. 95.

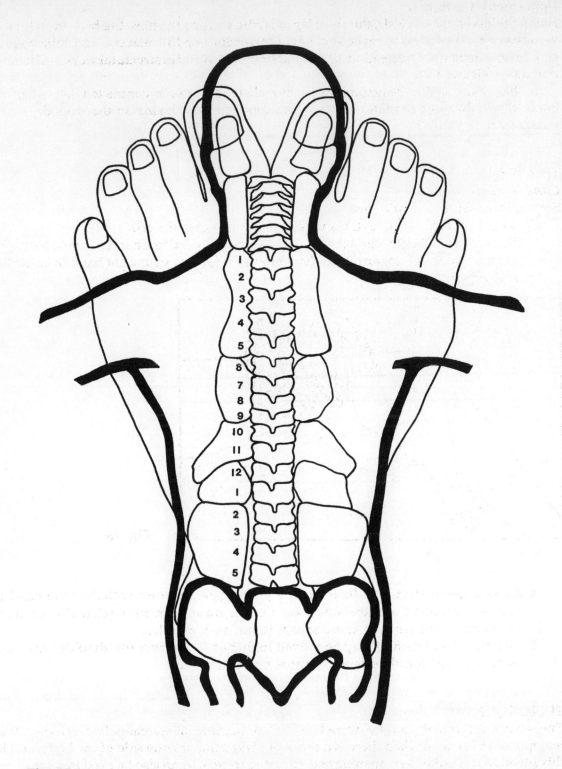

Fig. 95

Upper Body Corrections

Having released the os calsis, the short leg side, the sacrum, the hips, the back muscles and vertebrae, you now need to make some final corrections on the relationship of the head to shoulders and pelvis. The freedom of the diaphragm is critical in structural work — if it is not free now, release it!

At this point in the structural work our client still has a contracted left side, but interestingly the high shoulder side has changed and is now also on the left side, so we would treat as follows:

TECHNIQUE 1

Client is on his front

Step 1. Stand at the client's head.

   2. Turn his head to the high shoulder side, in this case the left.

   3. Place your left hand behind the left ear over the temporal bone and occipital base. The air, fire and water fingers fit neatly over this area. Place your right hand over the left scapula (Fig. 96).

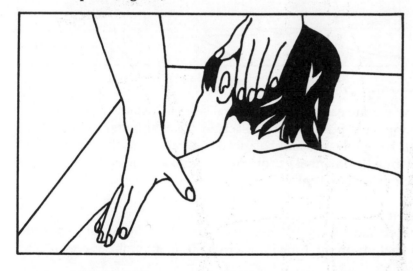

Fig. 96

   4. Apply a gentle stretch to the tissues by pushing gently down with the right hand as you gently pull the left hand towards you. This is a straight line stretch. Do not rotate the head as this tends to cause spasm in the neck muscles.

   5. The right-hand contact may be moved higher or lower over the shoulder area and close into the dorsal vertebrae on that side if indicated.

TECHNIQUE 2

The above treatment can be varied so as to become a cranial-pelvic release. This manipulation is useful when there is a sense of contraction on one side of the body, and in this situation it is done as an opening and releasing stretch. It can also be used in cases of ear trouble and as a release for the hips, as the innominates and parietal/temporal bones have a relationship through symmetry of form.

111

Client is on his front
Step 1. Stand at the client's head.
    2. Place the air, fire and water fingers of your left hand over the temporal bone and occipital base, and your right hand on the left innominate bone (Fig. 97).
    3. Apply a slight stretch between your contacts and hold for 1 minute. If you feel stimulation is necessary then vibrate your contacts.

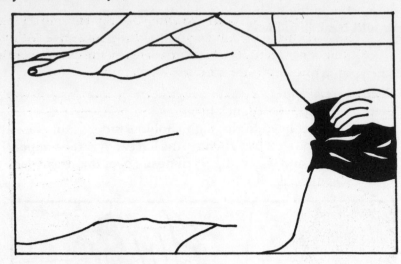

Fig. 97

TECHNIQUE 3. SACRAL-OCCIPITAL BALANCING

Sacral-occipital balancing can be done earlier in a structural session, usually after the point when you have finished working on re-positioning the sacrum. It can be better left to the end because by that time you will have released and balanced the structures that lie between these two bones, thereby clearing the channel of communication. Fig. 67 shows the direct relationship between the occiput and sacrum.

Client is on his front
Step 1. Stand at the client's left side.
    2. With the thumb of your left hand find sore spots on either side of the occiput, and with your right thumb find related sore spots on the sacrum. Remember the energy blocks

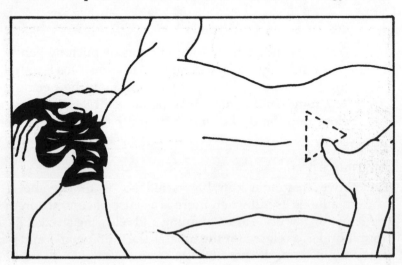

Fig. 98

often relate diagonally. Sore spots on the left side of the occiput may reflex to sore points on the right side of the sacrum (Fig. 98).

3. Stimulate alternately for 1-2 minutes until the soreness disappears.
4. Place your left thumb on a sore spot over the occiput and place the thumb of your right hand on the apex of the sacrum, with fingers relaxed on the buttock (Fig. 99).
5. Apply a gentle lift, and hold with your right thumb on the apex of the sacrum directed towards the right hip as you hold the sore spot with your left thumb.
6. Hold for 1-2 minutes. Feel for a sense of the energy coming in to balance, or it singing in harmony, to use a musical metaphor.

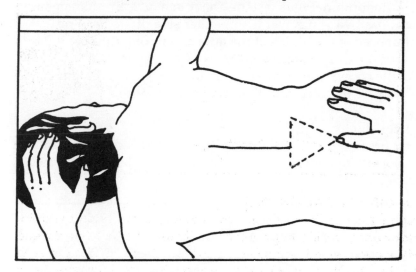

Fig. 99

7. Place your left hand palm down on the occiput, and your right hand palm down over the sacrum (Fig. 100).
8. Alternately stimulate the sacrum and occiput by very gentle vibration of your hands for about one minute. Hold and visualise the two bases levelling and balancing in relation to each other.

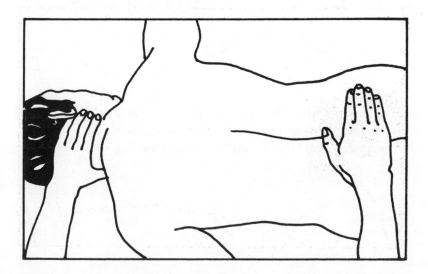

Fig. 100

113

Note: The visualisation that I use for this is based upon the kite illustration of the sacral-occipital relationship as shown in Fig. 67. I visualise, in my mind's eye, the two bones as triangles whose bases are offset in relation to each other. As I hold and balance I see them moving into a perfect relationship, bases matching exactly, creating the diamond or kite shape of normal functioning. I find this image a powerful focus for my intentionality.

TECHNIQUE 4. SPHENOID–COCCYX BALANCING

The sphenoid and coccyx are the two bones at either end of the spine. Their relationship is shown in Fig. 92. They are, respectively, the positive and negative poles of the spine and of the sympathetic branch of the autonomic nervous system. The sphenoid is a predominantly internal bone in the skull but it has two wings that lie on either side of the head near the temples, and it can also be influenced at the bridge of the nose as part of it runs behind the eyes. Due to the involvement of the deep diagonal currents of energy in this technique, when balancing the left side of the coccyx you correlate it to the right wing of the sphenoid, and vice versa, or polarise the tip of the coccyx to the bridge of the nose.

Client is on his front

Step 1. Stand at the client's left side.

2. Place the tip of your right fire finger on the left side of the client's coccyx and your left thumb on the right wing of the sphenoid, the fingers relaxed on the head or spread up and out like an aerial (Fig. 101).

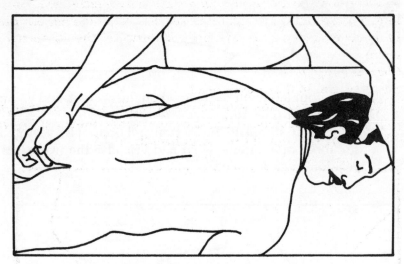

Fig. 101

3. Stimulate the coccyx gently with a small circular movement as you hold the sphenoid for about 1 minute. Hold and feel for the energy coming in to balance.

4. Alternatively you may place your fire finger on the tip of the coccyx and your left thumb on the bridge of the nose (Fig. 102). Stimulate as in step 3.

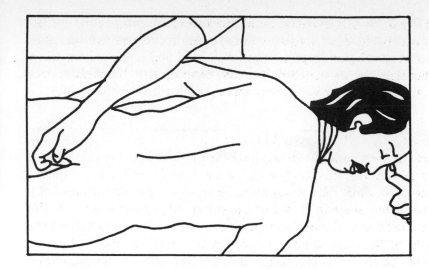

Fig. 102

TECHNIQUE 5. THE NORTH POLE STRETCH

This is a technique that is used to correct anterior vertebral curves and compression of the discs in the cervical and upper dorsal regions. It may be necessary to place cushions underneath the head and under the hips to correct any anteriority of the vertebrae before making this correction. The manipulation is done slowly and carefully. The client's body should be able to move freely on the table. This technique is not used on clients who have a long or loose neck. The technique can also cause momentary dizziness particularly in cases of poor circulation, as the body adjusts to the increased circulation of blood and energy.

Client is on his back

Step 1. Stand at the client's head.

    2. Place both hands behind the head so that you are holding the occipital bone with your fire and air fingers. The hand position is shown in Fig. 103. The thumbs are placed along the line of the jaw to firm the hold.

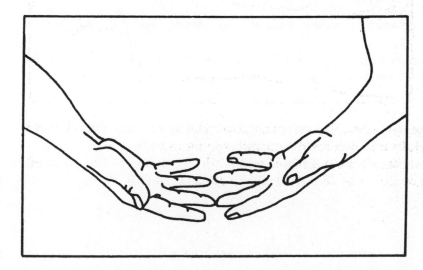

Fig. 103

3. Tilt the chin towards the chest and have the client take a deep breath as you hold the head under very slight traction. Have the client take at least three deep breaths. Allow time for a relaxation between each breath (Fig. 104).
4. At the end of the last out-breath, provided no pain or discomfort has been experienced by the client, a short corrective pull of half-an-inch may be given if deemed necessary.

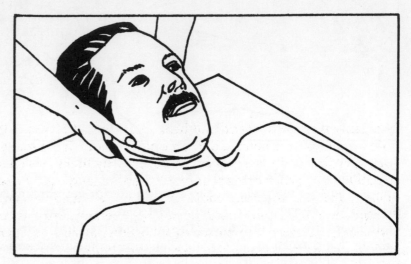

Fig. 104

After three sessions of structural bodywork incorporating all of the above techniques and other general balancing as well, the main changes in our client are, working from the bottom up, the sacrum is still not level, the tension in the left buttock is gone. The innominates are only slightly uneven. The shoulders are level and the arms are hanging more evenly. However, the major change is that the spine is now compensating naturally for the sacral distortion in that it now has a curvature to the right. What this means is that the layer of adaptation has been removed. The client no longer has the pain in the sacrum, though from a structural point of view only the first layer of imbalance has been dealt with. Further improvement is definitely possible and will no doubt occur in subsequent sessions.

As a final thought — and make of this what you will — if when you re-check a client at the end of a structural session there is no obvious improvement, or indeed if things look a bit worse, never tell the client. Always say that things are much improved. Be encouraging! You did not set out to make them worse and it is very unlikely that has happened, just that it is going to take a while for the changes to show physically. Do not project your own fears onto the client. Because most people's kinesthetic perception of their posture is faulty, they cannot tell whether what you are saying is true or false.

9 Self Help

In polarity therapy the term 'self help' refers to that aspect of the therapy which the client does for themselves outside of the treatment room. It is usually taken to consist of polarity yoga exercises and dietary changes. All polarity therapists should have an understanding and ability to teach clients appropriate exercises and useful dietary reforms. However, it is unlikely that any therapist could be said to be equally skilled in all of the four areas of therapeutic intervention used in polarity therapy. Most therapists will, apart from the bodywork, specialise in at most two of the other three areas, though they will be competent in all. My own work is mainly focused around bodywork, counselling and exercise. I do very little dietary therapy, just the occasional purifying programme and some other simple changes at most. Another area of self help is to teach the client specific energy balancing manipulations.

Polarity yoga exercise, or polarenergetics as it is sometimes called, is a huge area of practice. The subject really warrants a whole book in itself. I am going to confine myself to some generalised observations concerning its usage. One of the first things I realised after beginning to practise as a polarity therapist was that few clients want to spend any great length of time working on themselves. The basic attitude was to the effect that I will do it for a while if it helps but I really just want to get on with life again and not be bothered about this stuff. It can be difficult to educate clients to the need for self maintenance. Polarity yoga, fortunately, is effective when done for only a few minutes a day, though obviously the results are better if done for longer than this. Overall the biggest problem is to persuade the client of the need to warm up properly before trying the actual exercises. There is something of a tradition in the west of throwing yourself into an exercise programme without adequate preparation, exhausting and possibly injuring yourself in the first session and then giving up on the whole thing. If you are going to teach polarity yoga it is important to understand how to warm up and relax the muscle groups used in a particular exercise.

It is also vitally important to instil in the client the concept of 'mindful' exercise. Whilst many of the polarity yoga exercises are very dynamic they should never be done without a full body awareness. Without this it is so easy to injure yourself. I have a background of many years of experience both of western callisthenics and oriental martial arts. Through these activities, in particular the Chinese internal martial arts, I learned a great deal about people's attitudes to exercise, how to warm up the body before exercising and the concepts of effortlessness and mindfulness in relation to physical activity. I have always tried to teach the polarity yoga exercises with an emphasis on making the movements both effortless and mindful. One of the best ways to get these points across is in a group situation by teaching a polarity yoga exercise class. In such a class you can teach warm-ups, movement concepts and actual exercises with quite a different quality from that which occurs if you do it in an actual therapy session. The group situation is somehow less of a problem for people, in as much as they get to see that there is nothing unique in their inability to do some of the polarity yoga exercises. Psychologically this is a valuable experience in terms of their self image.

It is also important to realise that some of the polarity yoga exercises are extremely difficult to do, particularly if a client has led a very sedentary life style. For example, in this sort of scenario it is very unlikely that a client would be able to get their feet flat on the floor in the squatting position. This kind of difficulty is often due to tension in the muscles surrounding the hip and ankle joints. It can require a long period of gentle stretching and muscle activation before a full squat is possible, in which case teaching simple variations of the squat is valuable, as is showing how to use aids to facilitate the attainment of the position. Putting a number of heavy books underneath the heels is one of the simplest aids to doing the squat. If it is practised on a daily basis the thickness of the books can be reduced every week or so as the flexibility increases until the feet are finally flat on the floor. Do not let your clients force themselves in to the final position in any exercise if doing so causes any discomfort other than a sense of stretch in the tissues. Pain is a contra-indication in any exercise. It is an invitation to serious injury.

There is a great deal of room for creative modification of the classic polarity yoga exercises as systemised by Dr. Stone. One area that is certainly worthy of a great deal of thought is that of combining the exercises into flowing sequences of movement that perhaps move through the cycle of the elements or through the structure of the body in a sequential fashion. It would not seem to be beyond the bounds of possibility to create some hand múdras to go with the movement sequences, made up of gestures that are in fact reflex release techniques. At the moment I know that many experienced therapists are seriously looking at the whole area of combining exercises with reflex release work with a view to making this a cohesive approach.

When working with a client on dietary changes the main point to bear in mind is the kind of mental emotional attachment that people can get to food. In many cases it has come to mean far more to the client than simple body sustenance, and the emotional satisfaction of fulfilling a basic need with a good meal. It often becomes a substitute for emotional nourishment, due to their inability to form stable intimate relationships or as a way of dealing with their feelings and emotions through the energetic changes that eating creates. Fundamentally, eating diverts your fire energy to your digestive system so people who eat too much are often suppressing their vitality, sometimes because they have a basic inability to focus their energy in any particular direction. I have found that getting a client to fast for as little as one day is an excellent way of highlighting the particular emotional reactions that they have to food.

I suspect that few people have a balanced attitude towards their diet. Over the last few years I have noticed that virtually every popular magazine or newspaper has at sometime or another run a nutritional advice column or a series on nutrition and diet. The problem is that all the so-called experts disagree. It is also true that at any time during the year you will find a book on diet and nutrition in the best sellers list. High fibre diets have been 'in', raw food diets, Beverly Hills diets, the anti-cellulite diet, the list is endless and ultimately most if not all of these diets are unbalanced in some way or another. The truth is, any change in your diet will produce some kind of change in your body, beneficial initially. It is when people stick to them rigidly that problems occur. I believe there is an innate fundamental wisdom in the body that will tell you what kind of diet you should eat at any one time. That same wisdom will modify it when necessary. Sadly, for most people there has to be quite a lot of mental-emotional and energetic balancing for this process to be able to function properly, due to the incredible amount of conflicting information that is constantly thrust at us.

I have worked with many clients over the last few years suffering from different kinds of cancerous conditions. During this same period there has been an enormous amount written on the relationship between diet and cancer, both from the point of view of a poor diet being a causative factor and a good diet being a powerful remedial therapy. I noticed that many clients had taken this idea on board, to the extent that not only did they feel that their diet was a causative factor but they had also become truly obsessive about their new 'healthy' organic, vegan, wholefood regime. I am not saying that such a diet is, in itself, anything other than beneficial in such cases, but I do question the powerful obsessive attitude that people often develop towards it as being anything other than a negative stress factor.

On the basis of these and other experiences I finally came to teach what I call the common sense approach to diet. Whilst I do not often recommend major dietary reform to clients I do spend a lot of time counselling them in relation to their attitudes about their diet. What I have found is that, firstly, the whole subject becomes less charged for the client, and secondly, that they change their diet according to their own intuitive sense of what is right for them at any particular time. I call it the commonsense approach because that is basically what it is. If you see a food product label showing that it is full of chemicals then it does not make a lot of sense to eat it. Unless you want to preserve your body for posterity! I suspect it is also true that if you have lived on a junk food diet for most of your life an instant massive change in your diet is not a good idea. It will probably make your body detoxify at a rate of knots, but in the long run my own feeling is that the time required for your body to change and learn to produce the right balance of enzymes necessary to process a totally different diet is years rather than months or weeks.

I am also fairly certain that there are some people who are now probably genetically incapable of being healthy on, for example, a vegetarian wholefood diet. In fact the genetic factor in diet is something that I have not seen explored in any depth. Anthropologically speaking, in any continental area there are usually races that are predominantly carnivorous and those who are mainly vegetarian. The indigenous Indian inhabitants of North America are a case in point. Some tribes were nomadic hunters who lived mainly on a meat diet, and some were farmers who lived mainly on grain and vegetables with a small meat supplementation. The inability of these and other races to handle the effects of alcohol is also a genetic factor in their constitution. Considering that at this stage in world history we are all quite mixed genetically, it is fascinating to realise that you can still easily spot people with a lot of Celtic or Scandinavian blood in their genetic makeup. It is also possible to recognise many others — yet another consideration when suggesting appropriate dietary changes, as if there were not enough already.

The other point about dietary reform is that, without doing any dietary counselling at all, clients will often spontaneously change their diets as a result of a series of energy balancing sessions. The better balance of energetic functioning seems to activate the innate wisdom of the body at a sub-conscious level. The client simply loses the urge to eat certain foods and also modifies their intake. Not that any of the aforegoing should give you the impression that you can ignore studying the dietary aspects of polarity therapy. There are some conditions that require fairly major dietary reform to effect a resolution, arthritis being one example.

However, I do feel that there is an optimal time for introducing dietary changes. It is important to remember that there is always a fundamental stress involved in any illness, and to insist on dietary changes immediately is often to add to that stress.

The other aspect of self help is to teach the client specific energy balancing manipulations that they can do on themselves. Many of the polarity yoga exercises incorporate specific release techniques, but to teach the client manipulations to do separately from the exercises can be of greater value particularly if they have some difficulty in doing the basic postures. When doing energy balancing on yourself it is important to build up the energy in your hands, or in some other way stimulate the body (which is the benefit of combining manipulations with exercise) before actually applying the techniques to yourself.

To energise the hands simply rub them together vigorously stimulating both front and back, then flick the hands as if throwing off droplets of imaginary water keeping the wrists and elbows relaxed. Place the fingertips together in a praying position and then move the hands circularly in a vertical plane that draws small circles at right angles to the front of the chest. After a few moments allow the hands to come to rest and separate them slowly until they are about five inches apart. Then move them back and forth towards each other with a small movement of no more than half an inch, until the unmistakable sensation of a field of life energy is experienced which is commonly felt as a sense of magnetic attraction or repulsion. At this point the hands are sufficiently energised to effectively manipulate the energy flow elsewhere in the body. It is possible to teach a client to do an enormous range of manipulations limited only by range of movement of the arms. For example, a five-pointed star release from the right hip to left shoulder can be done by placing the right hand across onto the left shoulder and working down into the pelvic muscles near the right Poupart's ligament with the fingers of the left hand. Due to the limits of flexibility of the hand, the left hand probes into the pelvis with the hand curled so that it is palm upwards. This technique works best with the knees bent and feet flat on the floor, as this favours the relaxation and release of the muscles in the pelvis. It is possible to teach a client to do nearly all the manipulations that you as a therapist perform on the front and sides of the body, from nine zone reflex release work to the perineal treatment. Techniques done on the back of the body can be taught with certain modifications, such as using the back of the hand instead of the palm and applying them whilst lying on the side instead of face up. The simplest way to learn how to teach these is to practise them on yourself.

A very simple exercise that can be done as the hands are placed in different positions on the body is to lie face up on the floor with the legs apart, and rotate them in so that the toes nearly touch and then out again repeatedly to a comfortable rhythm that is easy to maintain. This effectively activates the five bi-lateral long line currents of energy and the pelvic energy, in particular the sacrum which then through the six-pointed star stimulates the head and thereby all the major poles of the body. For example, another version of the five-pointed star release can be done by placing the hands palm down as described earlier whilst moving the legs for a couple of minutes, and then relaxing and feeling for the energy release. Many other techniques can be done in this way with the leg action stimulating the energy and the hands directing and balancing it.

You can teach your clients to do either specific manipulations that will support the treatments that you are giving them, or more general balancing techniques. I have noticed that some clients actually prefer doing this kind of work because it is easier than polarity yoga exercise.

A final aspect of self help that I use is the concept of 'homework'. All self help is in a sense work done at home, but what I mean in this instance by homework is getting an agreement from the client to do certain things outside of the diet, exercise and energy balancing areas. The kind of things I am talking about range from getting a client to do one self-indulgent act every week, to visiting the grave of a deceased relative. My own belief in the value of this kind of work comes from my own personal experience. Many years ago, when I was ten years old, my parents separated and I had no further contact with my father for some eight years. At this point I made the decision to go and visit him to say 'In case you are interested, I am your son.' One week before I was due to go and visit him the news reached me that he had died of liver failure due to alcoholism. This left me with a great deal of unfinished business. I felt full of anger and grief. Some ten years later, having done seemingly endless therapy on the issues with therapists who used every approach from Transactional Analysis and Gestalt to body orientated therapy, the anger and grief were still not resolved. During all the time since the funeral I had never visited his grave nor had any desire to. However, one day I happened to be in the vicinity of the churchyard where he was buried and on a whim decided to visit it. When I got there I found there was no head-stone to mark the grave, nothing to indicate that he had ever lived, which made me feel sad and tearful. After a few minutes I turned and headed back towards the car, and halfway there, literally in mid stride with one foot in the air, I froze because in that instant I knew that I had forgiven him, and all the grief and anger vanished. Now, I know it could be argued that all the therapy I had undergone had created the possibility for forgiveness to occur but the real key was the actual visit to his grave, and somehow if I had done that earlier I know the issues would have been resolved much sooner.

Since that time I have tested out the idea, when doing therapy with clients who are stuck with unresolved grief, that in some way visiting the grave is a critical action. In some cases I have even visited the grave with them. In all the cases where I have used this approach it seems to have marked a major turning point in the therapeutic work. This led me on to the whole idea of the therapeutic effect of certain actions in relation to a client's problems. A client with problems relating to their self-worth can be shifted quite dramatically by getting them to do one particular action that somehow is fundamentally meaningful and relevant to the quality of their self-image. The skill lies in ascertaining what action they need to undertake. Unfortunately, I cannot offer any real guidelines on how to choose the appropriate action. The process for me is an intuitive perception based on a deep connection with the client's energy.

10 Afterthoughts

Dr. Stone often compared polarity therapy to homeopathy in that the basis of polarity is 'like cures like' (*similaris curantur similaris*), a concept that is common to many systems of alternative medicine. In classical homeopathy, when an effective remedy is found the client continues to take the same remedy until it creates no further change in their state of health. At this point if they are not completely balanced and healthy again their whole state is re-evaluated and a new remedy prescribed. This same issue is raised when you have given a client a session that has had a great deal of impact on their energetic balance. During the next session do you by and large repeat the same treatment, or do you immediately follow up any new developments that have been created in their energy field?

The clearest way to illustrate this concept is to take the example of a client with an air elemental imbalance. In the first scenario you give them whatever kind of work that you feel is appropriate to resolving the air imbalance they are manifesting. At the next session you find that the treatment you gave previously had a good effect and that the air imbalance had resolved itself, but that they are now manifesting some degree of fire disturbance, so you treat the fire imbalance in whatever fashion you deem appropriate. At the third session you find that air and fire are now clear but that some other imbalance is showing, so you treat that and so on until all the energetic imbalances are clear and the client is healthy again. This particular way of approaching treatment could simply be called 'following the blockages'. In the second scenario the client is again treated appropriately for the air imbalance; but at the second session, rather than following the blockages you give them exactly the same treatment as in the first session. You would keep repeating the same treatment for as long as it continued to create change, and only shift to treating whatever energetic imbalance was manifesting at the point that the original treatment made no difference to the client's energetic balance. You would then repeat this new treatment until it created no further change and so on until the client was healthy. This kind of approach to treatment could be called 'repeating effective balancing'. Indeed these two concepts can be explored during a single session. Following the blockages during a single session would mean that you would not stay with a particular balancing approach if at some point in the treatment the client suddenly began manifesting other signs. This might lead you to change your treatment, say from working with the air element to working on earth, or you could ignore the signs of earth imbalance and continue with the air treatment.

Having used both approaches over a number of years I cannot really say that one way is superior to the other, but if I had to choose I would probably go for repeating effective balancing as my overall approach. Using this particular approach does not mean I only ever do one treatment on a client. In fact, in some sense all treatments are different even if you use exactly the same manipulations, but I am utilising a technique which by virtue of the client's own responses has proven to be effective therapy. In following the blockages I have come to the conclusion that the human energy system is a very subtle mechanism that is quite able to give you false leads, because as energy releases it will show up a multitude of apparent blockages and disturbances as the system balances and regulates itself. It is important to bear in mind that our energy system is self-regulating and will manage to rebalance itself very well as long as you simply maintain an overall impetus.

One of the first things I do after I have given a session, is to self reflect on my feelings about it. The sort of questions I ask myself are: how clearly did I see the client's problems? was it an effective session? how relaxed was I? did I tune in to the energy as well as I could have? what did I learn? did the client learn anything? what direction should any future therapy take? was the session an enjoyable experience? The answers to these questions and many others are not as important as the process of self reflection on the issues raised. If you are going to learn from the experience of giving a polarity session then there must be a period of integration, a time during which you evaluate the quality and content of the experience and allow this to modify your beliefs about and understanding of polarity therapy. This is essential if you are going to improve as a practitioner. Ultimately, if you do not grow and expand in your knowledge, the work you do will become rigid and it will not be long before all the heart has gone out of it.

One of the most interesting experiences that I have had as a polarity therapist is that in spite of the fact that polarity is a very powerful healing system in the physical sense, I have often treated clients who did not improve physically and yet who insisted that they felt 'healed'. Clients who were still in fact experiencing a significant degree of physical pain. The alleviation of physical pain was one of my early criteria for judging the effectiveness of my treatments. It took a number of these experiences before I realised something that is fundamental to my practise and teaching of polarity therapy: this is that health is neither the absence of physical or mental dis-ease nor the experience of continuous physical and mental wellbeing. Health is in fact all of these things. It is very simply the ability to change fluidly from one state of being to another. Health is an endless flow of changes. Most of us have a concept of health that is static. You are either healthy or sick. When the reality is healthy or sick you are still experiencing the continuum that is 'HEALTH'.

My clients' belief in a static concept of health created an interesting problem in terms of their continuing to use polarity therapy as a form of treatment. What their belief did was to prevent them coming to see me if they became ill after their initial course of treatment. Once their health problem had been resolved they somehow felt that they were not supposed to get ill once more. They then experienced a strong sense of themselves as being a failure if they did, nor did it make any difference whether or not the nature of the disease was the same as the original problem. I had originally thought that they did not return to see me when they felt bad again because they saw my treatment as a failure. I only discovered the truth of the situation because my practice was in a relatively small town where I would often meet my clients casually in the street. I would naturally ask how they were. It was then I discovered that they were often still having problems but had felt unable to come and see me because they thought they were not supposed to get ill again. They felt they had failed. What this made me realise is that I really had to explore quite deeply with them their basic concept of health, and get them to see it as a state of constant change; like a wave-form, there would always be highs and lows but the main thing was to simply go with the flow. If you are ill this week you probably will not feel the same in two weeks' time. You could be better or worse but ultimately all that was certain was that it was going to be different. For most of them such a dynamic concept of health was a real healing in itself. They no longer had to experience the insidious fear that when they became ill it was a sentence of doom that was perhaps going to define the rest of their lives.

A shift in a client's beliefs from health as a static condition of wellbeing to health as a dynamic process of constant change is the release of an energy block in the mind. This then allows the body state to undergo a change. It is worth realising that any belief that is fixed and does not admit or allow the possibility of change is a definite blockage to the free flow of energy in your body and your life in general. Some of my afterthoughts and reflections upon my experiences as a polarity therapist were that clients always changed but often did not get physically better. There was always a sense that the change was in their minds, or more specifically their beliefs, which nearly always created a shift in their emotions. Sometimes this was accompanied by a change in their physical state, sometimes not. Either way it did not seem to matter to them. Many times clients have said to me 'I came here for you to sort out my body and what you have done is sort out my mind', and yet gone away perfectly happy with this as a therapeutic outcome, even though basically this was not within the confines of the therapeutic contract.

This ultimately led me to throw out the idea of a therapeutic contract except in its simplest form, because it seemed that neither I nor the client was able to judge what the outcome of the work we did was supposed to be. Any kind of specific contract seemed to be a form of limitation. I have considered that if I do have a contract, what it says is 'create change and trust the life energy. It always knows best'. It seemed as time went on that I did not use 'therapeutic interventions'. What happened in a session was that my energy had a relationship with the client's energy and that 'something happened'. What this was, was never clear until later, but it was always appropriate. This was the beginning of my conceptualisation of the attunement approach to polarity therapy. This is not to say that I advocate this as an approach to take from your very first treatments as a polarity therapist. I think you need to start with some boundaries and goals so you can explore the vast possibilities that polarity offers and be able to make some sense of the responses you get. My approach could be described as being intuitive, but that intuition comes from years of study, practice and synthesis. I do not see intuition as having no form or structure as its foundation — quite the opposite in fact. The better the foundation, the better the intuition.

It also happened on occasion that clients got neither any physical improvement nor any mental-emotional change, or so it seemed. At first, I took these cases as my real failures, but I then realised that these clients were getting something else that I believe to be of definite value. What they got was an increase in their awareness both of themselves and of the people around them. An awareness of the nature of their problems both physically and mentally and what was causing them. Yet they were not going to try and change the situation. You could say that they were consciously aware of their ability to make choices and that their actual considered choice was to change nothing. I had often noticed that if a client did experience a major inner change, unless they supported this with an equivalent change in the outer form of their lives the change would not hold. The dynamics of someone's state of health is intimately linked with the dynamics of their personal relationships. I had noticed in many of these cases that it was the client's current relationship that was one of the major causative factors in their problem. This factor was often openly acknowledged in the course of treatment, and yet oftimes the client's decision was that for any number of reasons they were not prepared to initiate any changes in the relationship. This, of course, is a perfectly valid choice and the key word here is 'choice'. Choice based upon an awareness of the facts. There is also no implication in these situations that the clients' choices will not change at some point in the future. What they have gained during treatment is both awareness of themselves and an acknowledgement of their ability to choose the kind of life experiences that they have with all the implications, both positive and negative.

It has always seemed a rather difficult question to answer in the light of all my experiences regarding the possible outcome of a series of polarity sessions, to determine when the work was finished. Indeed, for some of my clients it seemed as though their decision was that it was never going to end. They were quite happy with the idea of having fortnightly or monthly sessions until the end of time. I personally found these clients extremely rewarding to work with, not the least because of the depth of relationship that occurred between us. This kind of scenario allows you to study the effects of polarity therapy on a much longer time-scale than is usual. It also allows you to practise polarity therapy as a preventative health care system and to do a great deal of health education. In many cases the end point of the therapy occurred when the client was finally free of pain. In other cases the situation was not nearly so clear cut and ultimately I had to rely on my own ability to recognise the point at which the therapy I was offering was not creating any further positive changes. This was not always a point of resolution for the client's problems, and so I found it essential to build up a referral system whereby a client was not left without any possibility of further change. I think it is essential in these situations to keep hope alive by giving the client a number of alternative routes forwards. It is also important to prevent the client from thinking that their problems are too difficult to resolve simply because your work with them was not fully successful. Do not be afraid to admit your limitations, particularly to yourself. Once again the need for education on the nature of health, and an unbiased overview of the many systems of alternative health care that are available, is useful.

The only real failures that I can think of from all the thousands of treatments that I have given were the treatments in which I could not connect with the energy. Sometimes this happened at the very first session, in which case the client often did not come back for another, no doubt saving us both a lot of wasted time and energy. At other times it occurred during the middle of a series of treatments, often at what I call the plateau phase in therapy. This is a place at which there is an apparent lack of progress but which in reality is probably a space for integration before new movement begins. When the therapy reaches this point it often breaks off for a while before you get a call asking for another session. A great deal of learning can take place for you as a practitioner when you feel that you have failed in some way. It is a wonderful opportunity for some deep self reflection on your own development as a therapist.

The practice of therapy should be a joyful, fulfilling experience, not a burden. If you do healing work because you feel you must, because you need to heal, or because you feel it is a spiritual obligation imposed upon you, then you are doing it for the wrong reasons entirely. It is true that most people become therapists because they have a need to be needed, because it makes them feel worthwhile as people. Thankfully, over a period of time the actual experience of being a practitioner and the reality of spending your whole working life ministering to the sick and emotionally disturbed tends to resolve the problem. At this point a practitioner either leaves the work and becomes something really fulfilling to themselves personally, like being a builder, or they continue as therapists, becoming far more effective because they have lost their attachment to the process and do it because it is fulfilling and fun. They are no longer caught up in putting on a performance of 'caring healer' or some other related role. Some people might question the usage of the word 'fun' in relation to the practice of therapy, but in answer all I can say is, 'is it really that much of a burden for you?'.

To practise as a therapist over a period of years or even a whole lifetime requires a continuing development of your skills. Without this you will ultimately become stale and begin working by rote instead of by a dynamic everchanging process of interaction with the life energy. There is always a great deal of talk about the healing arts. We talk of polarity as a healing art. Are you a practitioner of the science of polarity therapy or are you a master of the art of healing with life energy? It is probably true that every student of polarity therapy who has successfully completed a training course is a practitioner of the science of polarity. Their heads are full of reflexes, positive and negative poles, sacral distortions, enemas and purifying diets, squats and positive thinking, causes and effects. The shift from being a practitioner to being an artist occurs at the point when you can let go of the idea of doing therapy and have the confidence to allow yourself to simply 'be' with the energy. A definition of art that I have always felt at home with is that art is the expression of the momentary perception of truth through a particular medium. The truth referred to is not necessarily a universal unchanging 'Truth', but the truth of the artist's inner reality at a particular point in time. The medium through which we, as exponents of the art of polarity therapy, express our experience of truth is our presence, our energy. The shift from practitioner to artist is the transition from being earthed in the principles to allowing yourself to be carried freely by the currents of the ether. A master of the art of polarity therapy is someone who can take one single technique and subtly modify it to fit ten different situations, unlike the practitioner who must have ten different techniques.

In the end, it is not the system that makes the therapist but the therapist who makes the system work. No matter how good your training the shift into artistry comes when you can transcend the limitations inherent in it. For all students, the position adopted in relation to the superior knowledge and experience of their teachers is nearly always one which limits the full expression of their unique potentials. To use a well worn phrase which is none the less expressive of the truth of being a student, whatever you are studying: 'if you meet the Buddha on the road, kill him'. Having killed numerous buddhas, I can vouch for this as an essential requirement for the true fulfillment of your therapeutic potential!

Appendix I

The Theory Behind the Manipulations
in
Polarity Therapy — The Power That Heals

The general energy balancing session as developed by Pierre Pannetier has been criticised unjustly since its inception. Some practitioners have said that there can be no such thing as a general session. Basically this is nonsense. It is obviously possible to stimulate and balance the energy in the body in a generalised fashion. The actual manipulations in the general treatment are extremely varied and affect the whole energy field. As a point of entry into the bodywork it is very useful for new practitioners to use the basic format, particularly when faced with complicated blockages which are difficult to diagnose and treat. Having the confidence to put your hands on a client no matter how difficult and convoluted the imbalance is, is sometimes all that is necessary to begin the process of clarification. The general session provides a familiar format with which to begin. There are many different principles of treatment involved in the full session, so I will discuss each in turn.

OCCIPUT AND TENTH CRANIAL NERVE This is a lateral balancing technique in which the air fingers contact the vagus nerve, which is the major part of the parasympathetic nervous system. It begins a relaxation response in the body through the activation of the vagus nerve. The occipital contact can affect many areas. It is the positive pole of the sacrum and the motor release area for the eyes. Stimulating the head always has an effect on the feet through geometric reflex relationship (Fig. 106, page 136).

FOREHEAD AND OCCIPUT This is an anterior, posterior technique that encourages the flow of energy from front to back. It will again influence the feet and is a release of the fire element oval.

TUMMY ROCK This is a balancing technique that affects the fire element and the water element. It disperses any excess of energy in the pelvis. The right hand can be moved up to the solar plexus area, in which case it is, to use Dr. Stone's terminology, a stabilisation of the airy mind patterns and the feeling centre of the solar plexus.

INSIDE ANKLE WITH FLEXION OF FOOT This technique mainly focuses on stimulating the various reflexes around the inside of the ankle. The reflexes in question are to the rectum, bladder, womb and prostate. The technique also influences the head through geometric relationship. When a client is relaxed enough the foot flexion will always make the head move. If the head does not move look for tension further up the body.

OUTSIDE ANKLE WITH EXTENSION OF FOOT Basically the same as the above manipulation except that the reflexes stimulated are to the kidneys, ovaries, testicles and the valves of the colon. The extension or flexion of the feet helps to lift the reflexes to the surface.

MANIPULATION OF ANKLE This point has a definite reflex to the valves of the colon, the diaphragm and the top line of the shoulders, this last reflex being an activation area for the parasympathetic nervous system. This last reflex relationship is an evolutionary reflex (Fig. 105).

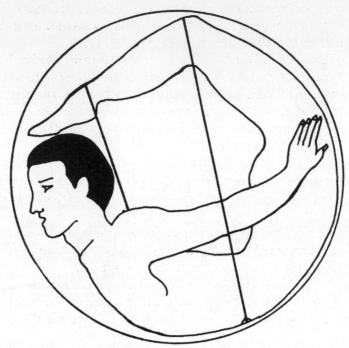

Fig. 105

TOE STRETCH AND TENDON COMPRESSION This technique affects the five bi-lateral long line currents of energy, thus influencing all of the five elements. It also stimulates all the reflexes in the feet and so influences the whole of the body.

TOE PULLS This is a tamasic technique which has a powerful tonic effect on the body. In a healthy person the toes are usually loose and will click easily on extension. It is possible that any one or all of the three toe joints may click. The tension in the toes and which joints click can be a useful diagnostic factor.

LEG PULL This technique is a specific adjustment for a high arch. It causes a gentle separation at the joints of the leg. The hand position on the top of the foot reflexes to the middle back. The technique can be done slightly lower on the foot with the middle finger influencing the cuboid, in which case it is a powerful stimulation of the kidneys.

PELVIS AND KNEE ROCK This is a balancing of the earth element (the astrological triad for earth is knees, bowels and neck), and will also free the hip joint which will in turn affect the ears and mandibular joint.

WRIST FLIP This is a simple relaxation technique for the wrist joint. The air and ether contacts create a diagonal flow of energy through the wrist in keeping with the idea that the energy flow crosses over at the joints.

ARM AND SHOULDER ROTATIONS Another relaxing technique, this time influencing wrist, elbow and shoulder simultaneously.

FINGER AND ARM STRETCHES This technique is the same as the toe pull and tendon compression, except that instead of working on the negative poles of the feet it influences the neuter pole of the hands. It influences all five elements.

THUMB AND WEB CONTACT This manipulation stimulates all the reflexes in the palm that relate to the organs beneath the diaphragm.

THUMB AND WEB CONTACT WITH INSIDE ELBOW REFLEX This is a reflex technique in which two reflexes are being worked together. It combines the hand reflexes to all the organs beneath the diaphragm with a reflex point on the inside of the elbow, to the liver and stomach, affecting mainly the fire and earth elements.

ELBOW AND LOWER RIB CONTACT This manipulation works by combining the digestive/abdominal reflexes that are located around the elbow with a direct contact over the organs themselves. This technique and the previous one use alternate stimulation, only one area being stimulated at one time, creating a 'push-pull' effect on the energy flow.

PELVIC ROCK This is a manipulation of the five-pointed star. It affects all of the organs lying on a diagonal line between the two hands.

ORBITAL CORNER AND OCCIPITAL RIDGE This manipulation illustrates the principle of working on a specific current line of energy, and in this case it is the ether current line. These two points reflex to the abdominal organs near the centre line of the body between the navel and the diaphragm.

CRANIAL BALANCE This is a lateral balancing technique in which each of the ten fingers tend to influence the corresponding current lines as they flow over the head. The anterior fontanel is a powerful point for creating balance in the body.

SENSORY/MOTOR BALANCE This is a final balancing of the sensory and motor currents of energy. The raised claw shape of the left hand will draw off any excess prana that has built up around the head during the treatment. It is also a release for the frontal bone of the skull.

CHAKRA BALANCE This balances the fiery life centre in the umbilicus with the third eye of the head. It balances the fire element and the fire principle.

FRONT AND BACK BRUSHING These last two techniques balance the energy on the surface of the body by connecting the therapist's positive hand to the negative side of the client's body, and their negative hand to the positive side. As the hands are moved down the body all the energy is balanced and any excess will be pushed downwards where it is grounded or absorbed into the greater energy field of the planet.

Having adopted many different approaches to the bodywork over the last few years I can personally testify to the quite astonishing effect a good general session can have on a client's energetic balance.

BALANCING THE THREE DIVISIONS OF THE NERVOUS SYSTEM This is a balancing of the autonomic and the cerebro-spinal nervous systems. In the upper contact the fingers affect the parasympathetic nerve reflex area along the top line of the shoulders, whilst the palm covers the sympathetic nerves on either side of the spine as well as the spinal cord. The lower contact also affects the three systems. The palm itself over the buttock line affects the parasympathetic nerve reflexes, and the fingers influence the perineal/coccyx area where the parasympathetic, sympathetic and cerebro-spinal systems terminate.

CHAKRA BALANCE The first part of this treatment involves drawing the five elements into the spine by placing the right hand palm up over the earth chakra (the palm up position is a hand mudra used in oriental meditation practice to draw in energy from the cosmos). The hand rotation over a chakra is used to encourage it to spin freely. The four lower chakras are balanced in relation to their supply chakra, the ether chakra, and then the ether and third eye chakras are balanced with the crown chakra. All the contacts follow the law of polarity, as the left hand is always kept higher whilst working on the centre line where the chakras lie.

BALANCING RESPIRATORY, EMOTIONAL AND SENSORY ENERGY CURRENTS This manipulation balances the chakras as well as the parasympathetic nervous system and releases the diaphragm. It uses sensory contacts (a very light touch) on the back of the body, the motor area. The contacts influence all of the five bi-lateral current lines. The upper contact points are along the line of the shoulders, which is the positive pole of the diaphragm, the air astrological triad and the parasympathetic nervous system. The lower contact is along the line of the buttocks, which is the negative pole of the diaphragm as well as being lateral parasympathetic nerve reflex areas, on the same line as the perineal floor.

GAS RELEASING TECHNIQUES These techniques would seem to be more physical manipulations than energetic, but remember that all matter is a reflection of energy so any coarse gases that are released as a result of these techniques are an indication of the release of a subtler vibration of life energy also. Dr. Stone seemed to use the term 'gases' in much the same way as practitioners of traditional Chinese medicine refer to 'winds'. For instance the Chinese refer to a headache as a 'head wind', and Dr. Stone also said that headaches were often caused by 'gases' trapped in the cranium (or sometimes by reflex pains caused by gas problems lower down). He felt that gases created by poor digestion could diffuse through the body and become trapped virtually anywhere, causing a great deal of discomfort. He pointed out that recurrent pains in the arms and legs could be caused by gases trapped in the haversian canals of the bones. The gas-releasing techniques are a treatment of the air principle in the body, the lungs being the neuter pole (the intake of air). The colon is the positive pole (a gas reservoir) and the calves of the legs are the negative pole. The effect of the various manipulations themselves is fairly obvious, but note that the second one is a seated diaphragm release. All techniques can be done including a gentle hold and sensing for the energy at the end.

UMBILICAL TREATMENTS The theoretical basis of these treatments is given with the procedural instructions. However, it is interesting to note that Dr. Stone called these treatments 'bloodless surgery without breaking adhesions', and felt that it was through these contacts that the primal energy of yin and yang that wove the body together in the womb could be influenced. I believe that in actual fact the umbilical energy centre (nabhi) is not synonymous with the fire centre (manipura chakra). In his early writings Dr. Stone refers to the fire element as relating to the fire chakra and the navel centre, distinguishing the two as different although later on he uses these terms interchangeably. I see the fire chakra as part of the caduceus system, the source of whose energy is the breath or prana. The umbilical centre I believe draws in a specific quality of prana directly from the energy that surrounds us all the time, that it acts much as it did in the womb, working fundamentally separate from the chakra/caduceus system. The caduceus is inactive until the baby is born and the first breath taken, and yet the umbilical centre is fully active where there is no breath and I am certain acts separately from the breath throughout the rest of an individual's life. The umbilical spiral links in to the physical body through the sympathetic nervous system.

PERINEAL TREATMENT The perineal treatment stimulates the muscles of the perineal floor. These muscles are the negative pole of the parasympathetic nervous system. It is the end point in the torso of the spiralling caduceus currents of energy, so it is possible to influence the functioning of all of the chakras and the balance of the autonomic nervous system with just this one treatment, which is probably why Dr. Stone says that it creates the biggest change in the energy fields of any single polarity treatment. Interestingly the whole of polarity therapy really grew from the perineal treatment, as Dr. Stone's first book was originally going to be a course on all the variations of the perineal technique. In the process of trying to work out the theory behind the effectiveness of this one treatment the whole energy theory of Polarity Therapy was born. When applying the perineal technique, if the pulse felt at the carotid artery is fast then you stimulate the area around the 1st, 2nd and 3rd cervical vertebrae lightly with the thumb and air finger of your left hand, as you hold the perineal floor with the fire finger of your right hand. If the pulse is slow then you hold firm steady pressure on the neck area and the perineal floor until the pulse normalises. As the parasympathetic nervous system has a powerful link with the chakras and the emotions it is interesting to speculate on the meaning of the phrase 'the seat of the emotions'. How many times when you were upset have you sat on your emotions to control them? As we literally sit on our perineal floor it seems there is some real physical meaning to the phrase and a fundamental truth expressed by calling the perineal treatment, to use Dr. Stone's title, 'mental and emotional therapy'.

RELEASING NECK TENSION (THREE VARIATIONS) These three techniques are different ways of working the ether element. The first two manipulations use the fingertips and opposite polarity of contacts to release blocked energy. The first uses an anterior-posterior release straight through the body, the second uses diagonal contacts through the centre (see also Chapter 5). The third manipulation polarises sore spots with a diagonal contact on the next oval field above to release the blocks. Polarising blocked areas in one oval field with the related areas in the oval field immediately above or below is a very effective treatment principle.

ETHERIC CURRENT RELEASE This treatment is in essence running the energy through a particular current line to clear blockages anywhere along it. It is an important treatment principle that can be used on any of the five bi-lateral current lines. All you need to do is adjust the hand positions to interact with the appropriate current line. For example, to run the energy through the earth current line all the contact points are moved out from their positions near the centre line (where they are on the ether current line) to points along the outside edge of the body on the earth current line.

TREATING BLOCKED ENERGY IN THE SHOULDER The first of the four manipulations in this treatment is a manipulation of the five-pointed star. The five-pointed star is an interference pattern of energy in the body. It is not a primary pattern of energy having its own particular source but occurs as a result of the intermingling of all the primary flows of energy. The technique releases the base of the star in the lower pelvis which frees the energy currents to the shoulder on the opposite side. The second manipulation is a release of the five current lines at the neuter pole of the diaphragm and the positive pole of the shoulders. The third manipulation (brachial plexus release) relaxes all the deep musculature in the shoulder area. As a treatment format for shoulder pain this works both the front and back of the body, but working the front only has a powerful effect on the back (and vice versa) through the concept of antagonistic muscular action, a physical concept which applies at the energetic level also.

KIDNEY TREATMENT This is a treatment of the kidneys by stimulation of the kidney reflex points in the feet. In the first manipulation the reflex point is stimulated individually and then stimulated in conjunction with reflexes to the whole middle section of the body, front and back. The second technique connects the reflex to the actual organ, and the third connects an air reflex point near the ankle (air astrological triad, shoulders, kidneys, ankles) to the kidney.

THE FIRE OF DIGESTION This is basically a treatment of the air element through the air current lines. Dr. Stone felt that most digestive trouble was not due to problems with the stomach, liver and intestines *per se*, but with the fact that the fiery fluids of digestion were stuck in their reservoirs and were unable to get out. He felt this to be caused by an emotional energy block in the air element due to emotional stresses diverting the impulse to movement. The air fingers and toes are stimulated so as to get the fluids moving through a general stimulation of the air element. The gall bladder itself lies approximately on the air current line and the first joint of the air finger is a specific reflex to it. The treatment is also beneficial in eye trouble and headaches, particularly when such problems are due to gas pressure from poorly digested, fermenting food. The eyes are the positive pole of the fire element and will benefit from the overall improvement in the functioning of the fire element, but the air current line also passes through the pupil and so this too is another factor. The jaw contact point is another reflex to the gall bladder and duodenum (the head placed in the chest area: Fig. 18, page 56, shows the jaw at the gall bladder level in the body). Specific indicators for this treatment are headaches, pulling and straining sensations behind the eyes, gas pains, abdominal cramps and excessive belching.

DIAPHRAGM RELEASE The diaphragm is a uniquely important muscle in polarity terms as it is at the middle of both the energy pattern of the five-pointed star and the interlaced triangles. It is the major neuter pole in the body. Its freedom of movement is essential to physical and emotional health. The first manipulation is on the foot reflexes to the diaphragm. The second uses the tibia release point on top of the ankle (see 'ankle manipulation' in general session, page 128) and connects it to the diaphragm. The third manipulation works on the long straight line currents at the clavicle line, which is the positive pole of the diaphragm and connects them to related points on the diaphragm. The fourth is a diagonal technique that stimulates the five-pointed star at the shoulder and along the diaphragm.

BRACHIAL PLEXUS The brachial plexus technique is designed to release energy blocks underneath the scapula that are adversely affecting the nerve plexus that lies in this area. This plexus is very important in that the cervical nerves from which it is formed are linked by rami communicantes to that part of the sympathetic nervous system that forms the cardiac plexus which controls the heart and lungs. It is an important technique for releasing energy blocks that are affecting the heart, which in polarity terms is where the air, fire and water elements are mixed. The shoulders are the positive pole of the air element and the brachial plexus is the motor pole of the air element in its respiratory and cardiac functions. In general the sicker the client the tighter the shoulder blades. The actual point to release is about one inch below the top of the scapula.

CRANIAL BALANCE The head is the positive pole of the whole of the body. This technique uses the air fingers as a negative pole when making the contacts on the positive head to create a balance. It is a lateral balancing technique. The treatment affects both the air and fire elements.

PELVIC RELEASE This treatment releases specific sore areas in the pelvis by using the left and right hands as positive and negative poles to push the energy through the blocked areas. I think of this as a 'pin point release technique' because the fingertips allow for a very precise release of small blocked areas. The technique predominantly influences the water element.

LYMPHATIC TREATMENT This treatment stimulates the water element in its function as the lymphatic system in the body. The techniques are done on the major areas of concentration of lymph nodes. It uses rhythmic squeezing to stimulate the flow of lymph and energy. The umbilical centre is used because of its fiery quality, which aids in fighting infection, stimulating activity in the lymph system generally and the elimination of toxins. In many ways the lymphatic system is the forgotten system in the body, and is only now receiving the kind of attention hitherto reserved for the cardiovascular and nervous system.

PROSTATE/UTERINE TREATMENT This is a perineal treatment (see page 130) used as a drainage release for the prostate/uterus. The contact area can be anywhere from the symphysis pubis to about the mid point of the perineal floor. The technique also uses related reflex points on the feet.

COCCYX TREATMENT This treatment is a balancing of the ganglian of impar with the cerebro-spinal function. The ganglion of impar is the end of the sympathetic nerve chain where it should polarise with the cerebro-spinal system. It is also a communication point between the right and left sides of the body. The technique affects the air, fire and water elements and also influences the earth chakra. The sphenoid/coccyx balance (see page 114) can be used after a coccyx treatment to balance the sympathetic nervous system.

COLON TREATMENT This is a reflex treatment for the colon. The reflexes that lie between the tibia and fibula are air element reflexes and relate both to the quality of movement in the bowels and the gases contained in the colon. The first manipulation is a stimulation of the air element by working the shoulder reflexes on the feet. The second stimulates the calf reflexes in relation to the shoulder reflexes on the feet and colon as necessary. The physical direction of movement in the second technique is with the anatomical direction of movement of matter in the colon, but is against the energetic flow in the calves, and so the manipulation is stimulating in its effect. Whilst the embryo is in the womb the reflexes are created by the imprinting of cosmic energy waves. Not only are air reflexes to the colon set up in the calves, but also fire reflexes in the thighs. The fire reflexes are a direct reflection (mirror image) of the colon in the thighs. The ascending colon has reflexes that run down the right thigh, the transverse colon is the knee area, and the descending colon has reflexes that run up the left thigh.

KNEE PAIN TREATMENT This technique uses the pinpoint release concept mentioned in the pelvic release. It uses the air and fire fingers to release energy blocks around the knee and activates the deep currents of energy that cross over in the joint by diagonal contacts. When a blockage will not release then changing the fingers often helps; i.e. putting the fire finger where the air finger was, and vice versa.

HIP TREATMENT This is a balancing by contour (see page 71). It releases the hips by polarising them with positive pole at the shoulders. It has a releasing effect on the diaphragm. Remember that all the major joints in the body have a definite reflex or polarity relationship to each other.

BACK PAIN TREATMENT The first manipulation connects spinal reflexes on the feet to the back (see page 110 for precise location of spinal reflexes). The second connects and reflexes to the back. The third manipulation again releases blocked areas by pinpoint release, using positive and negative contacts.

VERTEBRAE PAIN TREATMENT This treatment uses two diagonal contacts between the ether and air fingers on each hand. Every vertebra is a polarised cross-over point of energy waves. The right side is positive and the left is negative, and the cross-over is bi-polar from the positive right side above to the negative left articulation below it. The vertebrae above and below a sore vertebra are treated because it is these which are fixed and which throw an excessive load on the vertebra in between.

SPINAL TREATMENT This treatment stimulates the sympathetic nerves that run along either side of the spine. It also activates the ether current line. It influences the energy currents as they cross over at each vertebra.

LATERAL SPINAL BALANCING This simple technique balances the vertebrae laterally. Vibratory impulses can be used in specific directions to reposition vertebrae.

SHORT LEG TREATMENT This is a structural technique that repositions the sacrum. For further information on the sacrum and short leg, see Chapter 8 in this book.

SCIATICA TREATMENT This technique uses foot flexion to stretch the muscles along the back of the leg, and through the attachment of the various muscles to the hips the movement has a releasing and decompressing effect on the sacrum, its articulations and the fifth lumbar vertebrae.

Appendix II

The Hermetic Roots of Polarity Therapy

Any detailed study of Dr. Stone's writings on polarity therapy will reveal the influences from Chiropractic, Osteopathy, Ayurvedic Medicine, Naturopathy and Chinese Medicine. What is perhaps not so clear is the extent to which polarity therapy is based upon Hermetic principles. In his books Dr Stone mentions Hermetic philosophy and the concept of 'as above, so below', but a look at the seven principles of Hermetic philosophy will show that Polarity could as easily be called 'Hermetic Medicine'. The seven Hermetic principles are as follows.

The Principle of Mentalism

That the universe is mental, the All is Infinite Mind which is the fundamental reality and the womb of all universes.

The Principle of Correspondence

Whatever is Below is like unto that which is Above, and whatever is Above is like unto that which is Below, to accomplish the miracles of the One.

The Principle of Vibration

Nothing rests, everything moves and vibrates.

The Principle of Polarity

Everything is dual, has poles, and pairs of opposites.

The Principle of Rhythm

Everything has its tides, its rise and fall, its peaks and troughs; its equal pendulum swings to the right and left.

The Principle of Causation

Every effect has its cause, every cause has its effect, all proceeding by Law, never by Chance.

The Principle of Gender

Everything has its Masculine and Feminine aspects.

A simple reading of these principles should convince you just how much of polarity is based upon Hermetic principles. All are considered in some detail in Dr. Stone's writings, except perhaps the principle of rhythm in relation to energy flow in the body. This principle is certainly covered in great detail in Chinese energy theory, and so Dr. Stone must have been aware of it even if he did not write about it. Even more interesting is the fact that many of the charts are in actual fact re-drawn, modernised versions of charts created by Hermetic philosophers and alchemists of the sixteenth and seventeenth centuries. For example, the chart reproduced as Fig. 106 taken from the book *Polarity Therapy and its Triune Function* and entitled 'Chart 4. geometric, anterior and lateral polarity reflexes', is virtually identical to the chart (Fig. 107) created by the English physician Robert Fludd, during the early part of the seventeenth century. Fludd was a leading member of a group of medical mystics who believed that their work was the key to a truly universal science. If you compare the charts closely you will see that you only have to add three circles from Robert Fludd's chart to Dr. Stone's for them to be identical. In fact, looking at Robert Fludd's chart, the other relationships that it shows are specified in other places in Dr. Stone's writings as polarity relationships. For example, the circle in Fludd's chart that shows a relationship between the calves and the shoulder area is the anterior aspect of the air element triad or air principle relationship (chest, colon, calves).

Chart No. 4 Geometric anterior and lateral polarity reflexes as potent superior and inferior contact points polarizing the superior pole with middle or inferior pole.

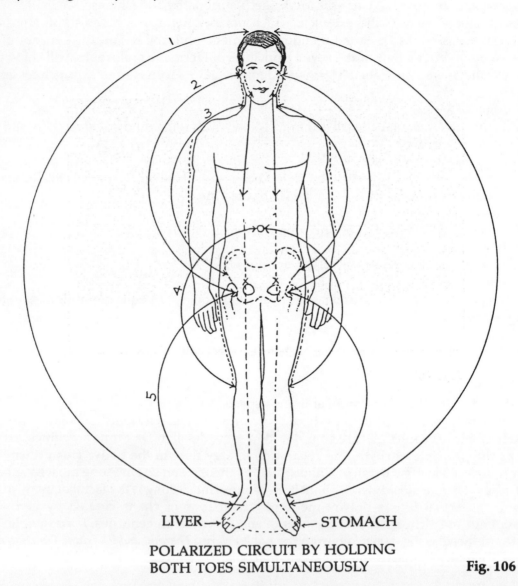

LIVER →   ← STOMACH

POLARIZED CIRCUIT BY HOLDING
BOTH TOES SIMULTANEOUSLY

Fig. 106

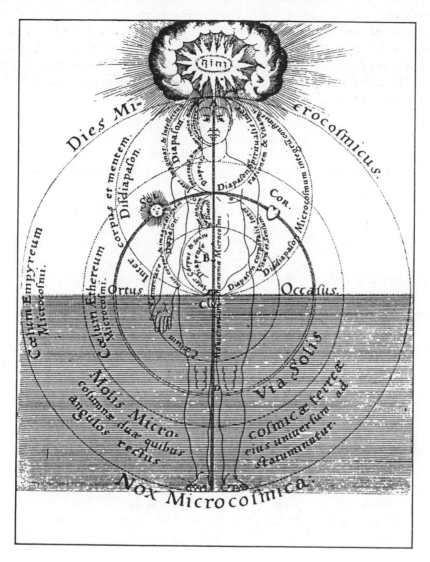

Fig. 107

Appendix III
Energy Models

It is an axiom that reality is far greater than the capabilities of our nervous system allow us to experience. The limitations of our language are also a fundamental impediment to expressing our felt sense of the subtler aspects of reality, such as the life energy. Having taught polarity therapy to prospective practitioners for a number of years, I am often confronted by anomalies and inconsistencies in the theory as set down by Dr. Stone in his many books and as synthesized by his successors. A guiding principle that I follow is that the map (or model) is just that and no more, or to put it another way a map is not the territory it shows or describes. Any time you work with a map or conceptual model it is essential to bear this fact in mind. If you do not then you are going to be limited by a false sense of its completeness, a feeling that it is the territory. This kind of belief, in what is essentially just one person's perception of reality, will radically suppress your creativity. A model structures your perceptions of reality. The more complex the model you work with the less freedom for unique personal insight and creativity, except within the confines of the parameters built in to it. Most people need models because they give a feeling of confidence and security. Problems arise when the model that they have been taught has been given to them as a 'complete' one. In this situation it is common for people to confuse the model or the map for reality or the territory. The simpler the model or map that you use the greater the freedom you have to modify it in the light of your own unique experience. Models and maps provide guidelines and a focus for your intention, and very little else. A map is ultimately just a guide to help you orientate yourself when you are exploring reality. If you are not prepared to alter the map in the light of your own unique perceptions of reality, then ultimately you will find that you keep getting lost.

It became obvious upon studying Dr. Stone's writing that his conception of the energy flows altered quite distinctly over the period 1948-1970, during which he wrote the books and supplementary pamphlets about polarity therapy. He always sought to improve and deepen his understanding. For example, his ideas on the construction of the gravity board changed between the writing of *Polarity Therapy and its Triune Function* (1954) and *Vitality Balance* (1957). If you study the text in these books in detail his concept of exactly what the gravity board showed and of the importance of structural balancing had also altered. His perception of the energetic function of the cerebro-spinal system also underwent a change between his first books, the *Evolutionary Energy Charts* (1960), and *Energy Tracing Notes and Findings* (1970).The point I am really trying to highlight here is that the polarity model was, during Dr. Stone's lifetime, always a model in transition. It is a tribute to the flexibility of his thinking that he did change the model over a period of time in the light of new discoveries and perceptions.

So, as a student of Polarity Therapy please do not get caught up in the model. It is neither the energy nor the body.

For Training and Seminars on Polarity Therapy throughout the world:

Contact Phil Young on

Tel: England 01392 215807

Email: masterworks@eclipse.co.uk

Web: http://www.masterworksinternational.com and
http://www.eclipse.co.uk/masterworks